THE DIVINE DIET

CAROLE LEWIS

Regal

From Gospel Light
Ventura, California, U.S.A.

PUBLISHED BY REGAL BOOKS
FROM GOSPEL LIGHT
VENTURA, CALIFORNIA, U.S.A.
Regal PRINTED IN THE U.S.A.

Regal Books is a ministry of Gospel Light, a Christian publisher dedicated to serving the local church. We believe God's vision for Gospel Light is to provide church leaders with biblical, user-friendly materials that will help them evangelize, disciple and minister to children, youth and families.

It is our prayer that this Regal book will help you discover biblical truth for your own life and help you meet the needs of others. May God richly bless you.

For a free catalog of resources from Regal Books/Gospel Light, please call your Christian supplier or contact us at 1-800-4-GOSPEL *or* www.regalbooks.com.

Caution
The information contained in this book is intended to be solely informational and educational. It is assumed that the reader will consult a medical or health professional before beginning this or any other weight-loss or physical fitness program.

Note
All testimonials have been provided to First Place by individuals and are based solely on their individual experiences.

Portions of this book have been adapted from Dr. Jody Wilkinson, M.S., *Health4Life* (Ventura, CA: Regal Books, 2002).

Cover design by David Griffing
Interior design by Stephen Hahn
Edited by Steven Lawson

Library of Congress Cataloging-in-Publication Data
Lewis, Carole, 1942–
 The divine diet / Carole Lewis.
  p. cm.
 Includes bibliographical references.
 ISBN 0-8307-3627-1 (hardcover), 0-8307-3717-0 (paperback)
 1. Reducing diets. 2. Weight loss—Religious aspects—Christianity. I. Title.
 RM222.2.L44595 2004
 613.2'5—dc22   2004026306

1 2 3 4 5 6 7 8 9 10 11 12 13 14 15 / 10 09 08 07 06 05 04

Rights for publishing this book in other languages are contracted by Gospel Light Worldwide, the international nonprofit ministry of Gospel Light. Gospel Light Worldwide also provides publishing and technical assistance to international publishers dedicated to producing Sunday School and Vacation Bible School curricula and books in the languages of the world. For additional information, visit www.gospellightworldwide.org; write to Gospel Light Worldwide, P.O. Box 3875, Ventura, CA 93006; or send an e-mail to info@gospellightworldwide.org.

CONTENTS

PART I: REALITY

PART II: FIRST STEPS TO CHANGE

PART III: THE FOOD CONNECTION

PART V: THE BALANCE

FOREWORD

Almost 15 years ago I was out jogging at a conference center in Florida. Hearing someone running behind me, I turned around to see a woman trying to catch up with me. This was my first encounter with Carole Lewis, but certainly not my last. As we ran, Carole introduced herself and told me about a program that she directed called First Place. She asked if I would be interested in speaking at a First Place conference.

I accepted Carole's invitation, and through the years since then, I have participated in many other First Place conferences. My work with First Place has been rewarding. The best part has been talking with men and women in the program. I will never forget meeting Beverly Henson after a conference in New Orleans and then seeing Beverly a year later—she had lost 100 pounds! What could be more rewarding than that?

As a professor of health sciences at Baylor University, I have devoted my life to studying the human cell and how it functions. In order for human cells to function properly, they must receive 45 nutrients from our diet. Not only do our cells need these nutrients, but also these nutrients must be consumed in their proper amounts. Too much of a nutrient or too little of a nutrient can be very unhealthy. In *The Divine Diet*, Carole Lewis has developed a complete and balanced approach that contains the 45 nutrients—each one in its proper amount. Following the diet plan provided in *The Divine Diet* will definitely improve the health of our cells. The reason we strive to be healthy and fit in the first place is so that we may serve Christ longer and better.

Richard Couey, Ph.D.
Professor of Health Sciences, Baylor University

A Fresh Look at Weight Loss

[1]diet n 1 a: food and drink regularly provided or consumed. b: habitual nourishment. c: the kind and amount of food prescribed for a person or animal for a special reason d: a regimen of eating and drinking sparingly so as to reduce one's weight. [2]diet vt 2: to cause to eat and drink sparingly or according to prescribed rules.

MERRIAM-WEBSTER'S COLLEGIATE DICTIONARY, ELEVENTH EDITION

When I say the word "diet," what pops into your mind? *Jenny Craig? Low-carb? South Beach? No dessert? Pills?* Or do you think, *What I eat for breakfast, lunch and dinner?* There is a difference.

Let me explain. Most likely, when you hear the word "diet," you think of one of the lose-weight-right-now regimens, methods or programs. Usually such a plan promises instant results if you drastically change what you eat or if you take some other dramatic action. Perhaps you have attempted at least one popular diet. Indeed, for many Americans, dieting has become an obsession—an all-consuming attempt to shed pounds and reduce the size of waistlines.

Some of the popular diet plans actually work—at least for a while. Therein lies the problem. When you complete the plan and return to a "normal" eating routine, the pounds return, too. Soon you turn to the newest weight-loss fad or the latest diet book. Thus, dieting becomes a cycle of losing weight and gaining it back, then losing and gaining it back again. Where are you right now on the lose-gain-lose-gain-lose-gain cycle? Let's face it: If the last plan you tried had kept off the excess pounds, you would not have picked up this book.

Most diets eliminate certain food groups, often those high in carbohydrates or fat, or those laden with sugar. Avoiding such foods can produce the immediate results you seek, but rarely do they lead to long-term success. Why? Because a particular food group generally is not the culprit. In fact, if properly prepared and eaten in correct portions, no food is really bad. God created them all: meat, grain, fruit, dairy products and vegetables. He even came up with the idea of fat! If banishing certain foods is not the key, then what is?

I suggest that the "secret" lies in looking at Merriam-Webster's other definition of diet. If you really want to permanently lose weight and improve your health, then you must begin to rethink the way you think about the food and drink that you *regularly* consume, not just what you eat when dieting. Moreover, you need to take a fresh look at how the shape of other areas in your life affects the shape you see in the mirror each morning. That is where the divine diet comes in.

DIETING THE DIVINE WAY

What would a divine diet look like? Well, for me, a divine diet would allow me to

- consume my favorite foods and still lose weight,
- dine at my favorite restaurants and still lose weight,
- pick foods from every food group and still lose weight,
- serve my family the same foods I eat and we all lose weight,
- get down to my lifetime goal weight and stay at that weight without changing the way I eat,
- know that my diet was never going to endanger my health, and
- be assured that my overall health would improve.

Sounds like a great plan, doesn't it? But is it possible?

I began dieting when I was 13 and have attempted just about every weight-loss formula ever conceived. A few of the attempts worked, but none of them lasted, until I was introduced to a Christ-centered health and weight-loss program called First Place. That was in 1981.

What I heard at the First Place meetings excited me. *Could I really eat from every food group and lose weight? Sounds divine!* I thought. *If this is true, then maybe I can stay on this "diet" for the rest of my life.* I learned that when you properly prepare your meals and eat moderate amounts, every food can be enjoyed. In fact, you will actually lose the excess pounds and become healthier than ever.

As I began to lose weight the First Place way, I found that I was beginning to look at dieting in a new way. In fact, I liked what I discovered so much that I am now the national director of First Place (sort of like Victor Kiam's purchasing the company that manufactures Remington razorblades because he liked the product so much). While most diet experts create a plan and then go about convincing you that it will work for you, I found a plan that worked for me (and works for others, too) and want to let you in on what I discovered.

LIVING IN FIRST PLACE

For nearly a quarter century, First Place has been the last "diet" for thousands of men and women. These people have lost and kept off their excess weight, but more than that, they have also discovered the rich and robust First Place way of living each and every day.

In First Place, we do not use the word "diet," because the first three letters are d-i-e. (Isn't that usually the way you feel when you are on a diet?) Instead, we call our plan Live-It.

As you read this book, you will come to see that the only divine diet is really no diet at all; rather, it is a balanced lifestyle that brings you health and wholeness. Balance is the key. When you learn how to balance not only your physical health but also your mental, emotional and spiritual health, you will obtain freedom and joy.

- *Physical balance* comes when you learn to enjoy eating healthy foods, not because you're trying to lose weight, but because the foods taste good and they make you feel good. Regular exercise is a vital key to physical balance because it improves your health while regulating daily stress.

- *Mental balance* comes when you learn to change your thinking about the foods you eat. Changing how you think will change who you are. This book will help you develop new ways of thinking, not only about weight loss, but also about who you are as a person.
- *Emotional balance* comes when you learn that eating certain high-fat, high-sugar foods will never fill the empty place in your heart. In this book we will face head-on your grief-causing behaviors.
- *Spiritual balance* comes as you learn to ask God for the help you need to lose weight and to keep it off. This book will show the divine way to achieve a life of spiritual balance, a life that is full of love, joy and peace.

GETTING A JUMP START

First Place is anchored in small groups that regularly meet in churches, homes and other places. A First Place group probably meets some place near you. Joining such a group and reaping the greatest benefits do take time, but losing weight and becoming healthy work well in such a setting because you become accountable to the group, to the leader, to God and to yourself. We emphasize connecting with other people while you transform your life because we have found that accountability is necessary if you are to succeed.

I can almost hear you thinking, *Ah, this all sounds great, but I am too busy. I do not have time!*

You are not alone in your plight and your fight to find the time. You want to lose weight and live a healthy lifestyle but you can't fit a program into your schedule, or perhaps joining a group just isn't your style. I hear you, and that is why I have written this book.

What follows is a jump start to losing weight the First Place way.

Here you have a quick scan of highlights and key principles that will point you in the right direction. If you embrace and act upon what I lay out, you will have taken important first steps and will see some immediate benefits. Many diets can help you lose weight, but what you will find in this book and in First Place will take you beyond dieting and lead you to living a healthy and whole life.

Part I

REALITY

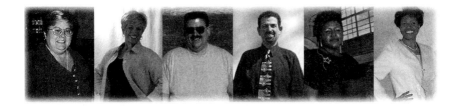

C h a p t e r   1

BROKEN DIETS

We did not dare to breathe a prayer or give our anguish scope!
Something was dead in each of us and what was dead was hope.

OSCAR WILDE

Though some details have been embellished for dramatic effect, the following is a true story. In fact, it could be about me, you or any of the 50 million Americans who each year attempt to lose weight.[1]

A cool breeze chased the sun toward the horizon and traffic slowed nearly to a stop as Andrea inched her way home from her part-time job at the local library. It was an afternoon like too many others: The 39-year-old mother of two teenaged boys had gone nonstop since breakfast, had skipped lunch, had grabbed a handful of M&Ms from the candy jar on her boss's desk and had not made plans for dinner. She was hungry. *A grilled steak soft taco would be nice,* she thought, as she diverted her car toward Taco Bell.

At the drive-through window, Andrea handed over $2 and change and looked into the bag to double-check her order. The steak taco was there but so was a steak quesadilla!

"This must be someone else's food," Andrea protested. "I cannot eat a steak taco *and* a steak quesadilla! You must take this back."

Andrea's remonstrations got her nowhere. The fast-food maitre d' told her to keep the bonus tortilla. "You might as well," he smiled. "We would just throw it away."

Free food! It was a dream come true for a hungry person—but a nightmare for an oversized one. *OK*, Andrea glibly reasoned, *I will drive home and give the quesadilla to my husband.* Did she heed her own advice? No, of course not. Instead, she parked her car and gobbled down all of the steak taco's 280 calories, 17 grams of fat, 1 gram of fiber and 21 grams of carbs. As predicted, it hit the spot. Andrea was reaching for the car's ignition key when, from inside the Taco Bell bag, the steak quesadilla called out her name. *No, no, no, I am not hungry now! I ate the taco and I am full,* Andrea tried to convince herself. *No, no, no,* she thought after each bite, downing the quesadilla's 540 calories, 31 grams of fat, 3 grams of fiber and 40 grams of carbs almost as fast as she had consumed the steak taco. Yes, yes, yes, with one spontaneous visit to the drive-through window she had done what millions of Americans do every day—she had broken her diet.

AN ALL-AMERICAN PASTIME

How many times have you done exactly what Andrea did, or something similar? I confess, I have. Breaking a diet is easy. Maybe it is the temptation of the free collector mug that "forces" you to buy the super-king-sized soft drink or the huge slab of cake (with ice cream) that someone else cuts for you at your coworker's birthday party or the sample donut the smiling Krispy Kreme attendant hands you as you enter the store (of course, you are at Krispy Kreme to buy donuts for someone else, right?)! Indeed, Andrea fits the American stereotype of eating right one moment and then violating every rule in the book as quickly as picking up a taco at the drive-through window. Do you fit the stereotype, too?

If you are an adult who lives in the United States, odds are that you need to lose at least a few pounds. More likely, you need to lose a lot. While the media emphasizes healthy lifestyles and we spend billions of dollars each year on health-related products or services, the number of overweight Americans continues to skyrocket. Currently, 61 percent of adults are overweight or obese, and the degree of obesity in children is also rising at an alarming rate. At any one time, the majority of men and women are trying to lose weight.[2]

> It seems the more we get obsessed with weight, the more we gain.
>
> —GAIL WOODWARD-LOPEZ, ASSOCIATE DIRECTOR OF THE CENTER FOR WEIGHT AND HEALTH, UNIVERSITY OF CALIFORNIA, BERKELEY

Starting and breaking one diet after another has become a national pastime. Finding the one plan, pill, recipe, book, gimmick, natural herb, secret formula or medical procedure to lose weight for good has become an American fixation. In our everyone-wants-to-look-like-a-model society, we grasp at whichever fad promises to offload our excess weight.

In chapter 2, we will look at some of the various trends and programs, but first let's face the reality of the scope of the problem. How did Americans get so fat? How do bad eating habits, a lack of exercise and all of our broken diets affect our daily lives? What is the price tag of obesity?

THE COST OF THE OVERWEIGHT EPIDEMIC

Everywhere we look we can see signs of diet mania. For most people, it is an individual effort to change the shape of his or her body. However, only when we step back from the mirror and take a look at some statistics, studies and reports, do we see the true magnitude of the problem and its full impact on society.

Billions of Dollars

To get an idea of how the craze for weight loss has permeated our society, let's start with a look at how it affects our pocketbooks. (At least that is one place we have succeeded in becoming lighter.) Here is SmartMoney.com's list of products and services that relate to dieting, weight loss and healthy living and how much Americans spend each year on each one:

- $12 billion on health clubs
- $444 million on health and diet books
- $5.5 billion on health foods and beverages
- $17 billion on dietary supplements
- $1 billion on commercial weight-loss centers[3]

Depending upon what you include in each category, these figures will vary. In 2004, Lidia Wasowicz, United Press International's senior science writer, estimated that Americans spend $33 billion to $50 billion each year on "pills, programs, products and potions, all promising a more svelte silhouette."[4] No matter how you crunch the numbers, it is clear that Americans spend huge amounts of time, energy and money attempting to trim down and live healthy lives. Of course, we do it because we want to look good and feel better, but we have an even greater need for change when we weigh the dangers that being overweight present to our physical bodies.

THE COST OF OBESITY AND CHRONIC DISEASES

Among children and adolescents, annual hospital costs related to obesity were $127 million during 1997–1999 (in 2001 constant U.S. dollars), up from $35 million during 1979–1981.

In 2000, the total cost of obesity in the United States was estimated to be $117 billion, of which $61 billion was for direct medical costs and $56 billion was for indirect costs.

Among U.S. adults in 1996, $31 billion of treatment costs (in year 2000 dollars) 17 percent of direct medical costs for cardiovascular disease was related to overweight and obesity.

—United States Department of Health and Human Services, Centers for Disease Control and Prevention

HOW GOOD NUTRITION, PHYSICAL ACTIVITY, AND WEIGHT LOSS SAVE MONEY

Nutrition

Each year, over $33 billion in medical costs and $9 billion in lost productivity due to heart disease, cancer, stroke, and diabetes are attributed to diet.

Physical Activity

In 2000, health care costs associated with physical inactivity were more than $76 billion. If 10 percent of adults began a regular walking program, $5.6 billion in heart disease costs could be saved. Every dollar spent on physical activity programs for older adults with hip fractures results in a $4.50 return.

Weight Loss

A 10 percent weight loss will reduce an overweight person's lifetime medical costs by $2,200–$5,300.

The lifetime medical costs of five diseases and conditions (hypertension, diabetes, heart disease, stroke, and high cholesterol) among moderately obese people are $10,000 higher than among people at a healthy weight.

—United States Department of Health and Human Services, Centers for Disease Control and Prevention

Health Perils

Overweight and obese individuals are at increased risk for physical ailments such as these:

- High blood pressure (hypertension)
- High blood cholesterol (dyslipidemia)
- Type 2 (non-insulin dependent) diabetes
- Insulin resistance (glucose intolerance)
- Hyperinsulinemia

- Coronary heart disease
- Angina pectoris
- Congestive heart failure
- Stroke
- Gallstones
- Cholecystitis and cholelithiasis
- Gout
- Osteoarthritis
- Obstructive sleep apnea and respiratory problems
- Some types of cancer (such as endometrial, breast, prostate and colon)
- Complications of pregnancy
- Poor female reproductive health (such as menstrual irregularities, infertility, irregular ovulation)
- Bladder control problems (such as stress incontinence)
- Uric acid nephrolithiasis
- Psychological disorders (such as depression, eating disorders, distorted body image and low self-esteem)[5]

These obesity-related ailments cost Americans and our federal health-care system billions of dollars a year.[6] If this isn't bad enough news, we learn from the *Journal of the American Medical Association* that "15 percent of 6-19 year olds (almost 9,000,000) in the U.S. are overweight, and that rates of childhood obesity have been steadily increasing since the 1970s."[7]

Obesity is something as costly to society as smoking, yet the government and private health insurers have done very little to reduce obesity rates, partly because politically feasible, cost-effective strategies have yet to be identified. This should be a wake-up call. Obesity-attributable expenditures will likely continue to increase unless something fairly drastic is done.

The Centers for Disease Control reports several factors that have contributed to rising rates of obesity among youth, including

- more hours spent in sedentary activities such as watching

television and playing computer or video games;

- availability of fast foods and the supersizing of fast foods that lead to diets high in fat and sugar;
- high percentage of both parents, and in particular, mothers working outside the home.[8]

As parents who love our children, it could almost be considered a form of child abuse when, because of the foods we feed them, our children are taunted and teased because they are overweight. It is time that we take responsibility for the state our bodies are in and begin doing something that will bring the needed changes to our lives and the lives of our families.

A CHRISTIAN RESPONSE TO OBESITY

The state of health in America is not hopeless. In fact, we need to look at these statistics and decide that we are no longer going to contribute to the obesity of American adults and children. We could start the trend of change for our country.

Men, women and children in every evangelical denomination in America today are in the same struggle to lose weight as those who never attend church. A 2004 article by the Associated Press focused on my own denomination, which, by the way, has been given the prize as being the fattest denomination of them all. In the article, Autumn Marshall, a nutritionist at Lipscomb University in Nashville, Tennessee, explained, "Most evangelical Christians don't drink, smoke, curse or commit adultery. So what do we do? We eat. While the Bible frequently condemns gluttony, it just appears to be a more acceptable vice."[9]

> Obesity is something as costly to society as smoking, yet the government and private health insurers have done very little to reduce obesity rates. This should be a wake-up call.

The article also cited a 1998 study by Purdue University sociologist

OBESITY IN THE UNITED STATES

Obesity in the United States is truly epidemic. From 1993 to 2002, obesity rates increased by more than 60 percent among adults. Approximately 59 million adults were obese as of 2002.

Since 1980, obesity rates have doubled among children and tripled among adolescents. Of children and adolescents aged 6–19 years, 15 percent—about 9 million young people are considered overweight.

Only about one-fourth of U.S. adults eat the recommended five or more servings of fruits and vegetables each day. More than 60 percent of young people eat too much fat, and less than 20 percent eat the recommended five or more servings of fruits and vegetables each day.

Despite the proven benefits of physical activity, more than 60 percent of American adults do not get enough physical activity to provide health benefits.

More than a third of young people in grades 9–12 do not regularly engage in vigorous physical activity.

Unhealthy diet and physical inactivity play an important role in many chronic diseases and conditions, including type 2 diabetes, hypertension, heart disease, stroke, breast cancer, colon cancer, gallbladder disease, and arthritis.

—*United States Department of Health and Human Services, Centers for Disease Control and Prevention*

Kenneth Ferraro. In that study, Ferraro found that church members were more likely to be overweight than other people. He analyzed public records and surveys involving more than 3,600 people. His conclusion: "Southern Baptists were heaviest, while Jews, Muslims and Buddhists were less likely to be overweight."[10]

Rev. O. S. Hawkins, president and CEO of the Southern Baptist Convention's Annuity Board in Dallas, has written a book, *High Calling, High Anxiety*. The Annuity Board oversees the health insurance and retirement benefits for Southern Baptist pastors and their families across America. Hawkins wrote,

It seems the secular community is sounding the alarm over the evils of obesity, but Christian churches do not seem to have heard the message. We're pretty good at avoiding alcohol and tobacco, but 25 percent of us drink six or more cups of coffee a day. Baptists definitely hold the heavyweight title in ministry.[11]

One of our First Place leaders, Jim Clayton, is pastor of Dixie Lee Baptist Church in Lenoir City, Tennessee (see Jim's full testimonial following this chapter). When I first met Jim in 1993, his church was going to begin a First Place class. Jim joined the class and told me that the Bible study was so inspiring that he was able to bring a series of messages from the First Place Bible study during the 13 weeks he attended First Place. Jim stayed in First Place until he lost 85 pounds and has kept it off for 11 years. Jim says, "First Place has absolutely changed my life. My weight and blood pressure are under control (no medication), the colon problems are gone, and my 'temple' has become a much more acceptable place for Jesus to dwell in."[12]

Today, Jim and his wife, Anita, still lead a First Place class in their church. They have learned a wonderful secret: If Christians will set the example by losing weight and getting fit, people inside and outside our churches will most certainly follow.

First Place can be an amazing outreach tool for bringing men and women into church who would never attend otherwise. When our friends and coworkers see the obvious changes in our physical appearance, they will want to find out what we're doing to lose weight. It is a natural progression for them to want to do what we are doing—whether it is attending a First Place group or getting a jump start, as outlined in this book—so that they can lose weight, too. Many men and women have developed a personal relationship with Christ through their involvement with First Place.

Try to imagine what would happen if every Christian in America began today to exercise and eat only healthy foods. The world would take immediate notice, and our Lord Jesus would receive praise and glory for the changes Christians make in their lifestyles out of their sheer love for God and their devotion to Him. Imagine how the money Christians now spend on weight loss could instead be given to win our world to Christ. Every believer taking seriously the verses that say, "Do you not know that your body is a temple of the Holy Spirit, who is in you, whom you have received from God? You are not your own, you were bought at a price, Therefore, honor God with your body" (1 Cor. 6:19-20), could turn the tide of the obesity epidemic raging in America today.

> On average, both men and women gained more than 24 pounds between the early 1960s and 2002.
>
> —*United States Department of Health and Human Services, Centers for Disease Control and Prevention*

One of the reasons I am writing this book is to share the life-changing benefits of the First Place ministry and how God has used this sound, proven program since 1981 to help Christians bring balance to the emotional, spiritual, mental and physical areas of their lives. An even more important reason for writing the book is so that, after we Christians do what we need to do, our friends, neighbors and coworkers will see the outside changes and want to join us to experience the same changes in their own lives.

The testimonials scattered throughout this book have been chosen because most of these men and women have been on the First Place program for a number of years. They have experienced victories and defeats while heading toward their lifetime weight goal. These testimonials were written by people just like you and me; however, the key to their weight-loss achievement is that they have learned the important truth, If you don't quit, you will succeed.

Success is in the process, not in the program. God knows where He needs to work first and it may not be in the physical area. He might need to bring some emotional or spiritual healing before weight loss occurs. Because First Place is a lifestyle program of balance, weight loss is not the only goal of the program. Balance in all four areas of life is the goal.

Despite our fixation on dieting, the headline in the August 2004 issue of *National Geographic* asks, "Why Are We So Fat?" The article exposes many facts about obesity, but boiled down, it points to some basic truths about our poor eating habits and overall health. We eat too much of the wrong foods, we do not exercise enough, and we do not address issues in other areas of our lives that affect how and what we eat.[13]

In chapter 2, we will look at some of diets and we will see why following these fads seldom brings about the permanent lifestyle change needed for lifelong health and fitness.

Notes

1. Jennifer Anderson and L. Young, "Weight Loss Products and Programs" (No. 9.363), *Colorado State University Cooperative Extension.* http://www.ext.colostate.edu/pubs/foodnut/09363.html (accessed November 11, 2004).
2. Jody Wilkinson, *Health 4 Life* (Ventura, CA: Regal Books, 2002), pp. 62-63.
3. Trevor Delaney, "Ten Things The Weight-Loss Industry Won't Tell You," (January 2003). http://www.smartmoney.com/consumer/index.cfm?story=tenthings-january03 (accessed April 2004).
4. Lidia Wasowicz, "Diets: Battle of the Bulge Beckons Many," United Press International (May 17, 2004).
5. A. J. Stunkard and T. A. Wadden, eds., *Obesity: Theory and Therapy*, 2nd ed. (New York: Raven Press, 1993), n.p.
6. M. Freudenheim, *New York Times* (August 29, 2003).
7. *Journal of the American Medical Association*, quoted in "Clinical Guidelines on the Identification, Evaluation and Treatment of Overweight and Obesity in Adults" (Bethesda, MD: Department of Health and Human Services, National Institutes of Health, National Heart, Lung, and Blood Institute, 1998).
8. Ogden, et al., "Research Facts and Findings, A Collaboration of Cornell University," (Rochester, NY: University of Rochester, and the New York State Center for School Safety, 2002).
9. Autumn Marshall, quoted by the Associated Press (February 28, 2004).
10. Kenneth Ferraro, quoted by the Associated Press (February 28, 2004).
11. O. S. Hawkins, *High Calling, High Anxiety* (Dallas, TX: The Annuity Board of the Southern Baptist Convention, 2003) pp. 43-44.
12. Jim Clayton, personal communication to First Place.
13. Cathy Newman, "Why Are We So Fat?" *National Geographic* (August 2004), n.p.

JIM CLAYTON

Pastor

Lenoir City, Tennessee

I joined a First Place group in August 1993. At that time, I was 42 years old, and I weighed approximately 255 pounds. Over the next few months, I lost a total of 85 pounds, which brought my weight down to 170 pounds. For the first time in my memory, exercise became an important part of my daily life. I began a walking program that quickly reached the point where I was walking three miles per day, at approximately 14 minutes per mile, six to seven days per week.

In September 1997, I had knee surgery, and I had to interrupt my walking regimen. It was a particularly discouraging time in my life. As a result, I began to nibble at some types of food I had been away from for four years. During the next two years, my weight climbed back up to almost 200 pounds. It was then that I remembered the commitment I had made to God when I started First Place, that with His help, I would never return to my overweight condition or my poor health.

Today I am back to my ideal weight range of 175 to 185 pounds—and I plan to remain here. I cannot begin to tell you about all that First Place has meant in my life. The program has helped me through some very stressful, difficult times as a husband, father, grandfather and pastor. Each Bible study has built upon the previous one, increasing my understanding of where God wants me to be and how He wants me to present His temple to the world.

I am a pastor. Experiencing success through First Place has enabled me to share with other pastors the need for us to set examples of leadership and commitment. It has also shown me the importance of presenting ourselves not only spiritually fit but also physically, mentally and emotionally whole.

In 1999, my wife, Anita, and I accepted the pastorate at a new church, and we took First Place with us. We have seen God work in the lives of many people in our new congregation, and we have used First Place as a tool to reach out to our community. As a result, several people who had not worshiped at our church are now involved in our First Place program. They had heard about what God was doing and they wanted to be a part of something that would change their lives. We often get calls from people who ask, "When does the next session of First Place at Dixie Lee Baptist begin, and can I join?"

God continues to use First Place to change my life and the lives of others.

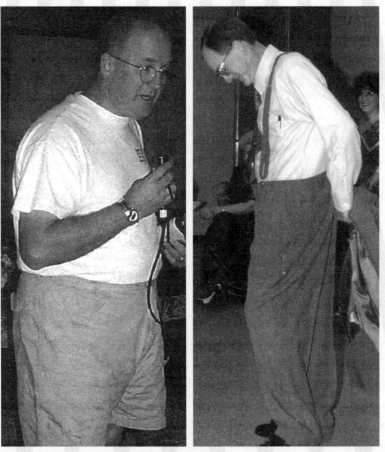

Before First Place   *Today*

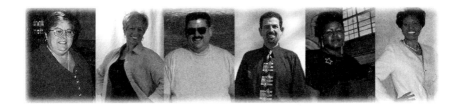

Chapter 2

TEMPORARY SOLUTIONS

I've been on a constant diet for the last two decades. I've lost a total of 789 pounds. By all accounts, I should be hanging from a charm bracelet.

ERMA BOMBECK

I giggle when I think about the diet I went on when I joined First Place. The rest of the class was doing the First Place Live-It plan—but not me. I was on a low-carbohydrate diet exactly like the one that has America abuzz today. I followed that diet because it was the last diet I had been on before I joined First Place. I lost the same 20 pounds I lost on the other programs, but I quickly gained them back. The low-carbohydrate diet worked because I had reduced my food intake to 1,200 calories each day, not because I was eating only 5 grams of carbohydrates.

Since the low-carbohydrate diet had worked once before, I decided I wouldn't bother to learn anything new—I would just repeat what was tried and true. I went through the entire 13 weeks of the First Place program, lost 20 pounds and never bothered to learn the Live-It plan. My group leader was so frustrated with my behavior that she recommended that I lead the next session—probably so that she could escape leading people like me!

All that has changed. I have lived on the First Place Live-It plan for over 20 years now, freeing me from ever having to diet again. The best news, though, is that I never experience the despair that followed when my diet of choice no longer worked. Because the Live-It plan is a lifestyle instead of a diet, we are freed up to eat a wide variety of foods. We lose weight by *healthfully* preparing and consuming *proper amounts* of foods from each of the food groups.

It is this memory of my own rebellious behavior that keeps me from ever criticizing any particular diet that catches the fancy of Americans. But there is much we can learn by looking at what works and what doesn't when it comes to trends. In this chapter, I will give you a brief overview of what I have found to be true.

POPULAR STRATEGIES

I have thought a lot about why we Americans, living in the land of plenty, are so determined to pursue one diet craze after another. Perhaps we feel guilty because we are overweight. Perhaps it is as simple as laziness—we want an easy quick fix, rather than a plan that will require us to revamp our entire diet and establish a regular exercise regimen. As Americans, we have literally tried everything from the grapefruit diet on one end of the spectrum to gastric bypass surgery on the other end. Let's look at some of the fads that promise people they can lose weight in a hurry.

QUICK WEIGHT-LOSS CLAIMS

Everyone has seen newspaper and magazine ads that make the most ridiculous promises. The truth is that these advertisers wouldn't be spending big money if people were not buying their products. Let's look at some of the claims and the truth about them.

While You Sleep

Losing weight requires significant changes affecting what kind of food, and how much of it, you eat. Claims for diet products and programs that promise weight loss without sacrifice or effort are bogus.

Lose Weight and Keep It Off for Good

The only way to keep the weight off after you lose it is to make permanent changes in how much you eat and how much you exercise. Be skeptical of any product that claims you will keep weight off by taking the product.

Mary Smith Lost 60 Pounds in Six Weeks

Don't fall for someone's claim of success. Who knows how Mary lost 60 pounds. She might be dying of some dreaded disease. It is physiologically impossible to lose more than two pounds of fat per week. Losing more weight than two pounds per week is actually a loss of water and lean body mass.

Lose 30 Pounds in 30 Days

As a rule, the faster you lose weight, the quicker you will gain it back. In addition, losing weight too fast may harm your health.

Companies spend billions of dollars each year, appealing to our appetites and contributing to our steady weight gain. In 1997, Pepsi spent $1.24 billion in advertising and McDonald's spent $1.041 billion.[1] By comparison, the Federal Trade Commission reports that all tobacco companies spent $11.22 billion on advertising and promotion in 2001.[2]

Losing weight isn't really all that complicated. We must reduce our normal food intake by 3,500 calories to lose one pound. A modest reduction of 500 calories a day will achieve this goal and we will lose about one pound each week. Reducing 1,000 calories a day will enable us to lose two pounds per week. If we have a lot of weight to lose, we could conceivably lose 100 pounds in a year, using this simple method.

THE SIMPLE TRUTH

The simple truth about every diet is that if it works, it is because the people on the diet are eating fewer calories than usual. Calories do count, and any diet that eliminates one or more food groups reduces calories consumed. "Diets that eliminate any of the six food groups should be considered fad diets."[3]

> Simply put, Americans need to cut down on caloric intake and increase their physical activity.
>
> —INDEPENDENT BAKERS ASSOCIATION

I have a friend on the low-carbohydrate, high-protein diet, and I asked her to tell me what she had eaten the day before. As she relayed every bit of food she had consumed, I was mentally counting the calories consumed the previous day. Even though she had eaten a fried egg and bacon for breakfast, a salad and chicken breast for lunch and a hamburger patty for dinner with another salad, she had consumed less than 1,000 calories. Anyone eating 1,000 calories a day is going to lose weight.

In First Place, the minimum number of calories a woman consumes is 1,400. On 1,400 calories of healthy foods, there is endless variety, and boredom is never a part of the process. Men and women who have a lot of weight to lose eat even more calories. The goal is to lose no more than two pounds a week, and if people are losing weight too fast, their calories are elevated until they lose no more than two pounds weekly. The First Place food plan is a balanced plan consisting of 20 percent protein, 55 percent complex carbohydrates and 25 percent fat. All food groups are eaten in the proper amounts needed to build strong cells while allowing us to lose unwanted fat.

The First Place weight-loss plan combined with regular exercise will lead to a lifestyle change that is permanent. The best part is that after we reach our weight-loss goal, we immediately begin to add more calories until we are no longer losing weight. Most women at their goal weight are able to eat more than 2,000 calories a day, and most men are able eat more than 2,500.

WEIGHT-LOSS SURGERY

Each year, more than 80,000 Americans are choosing surgery as a way to lose unwanted pounds.[4] Because gastric bypass surgery is only available to those who need to lose a lot of weight (80 pounds for women and 100 pounds for men) or who have a Body Mass Index of over 40 percent, it seems to many people to be the easy way to solve a complex problem.

Weight-loss surgery may be many things, but easy is not one of them. This is major surgery and "three in 1,000 die during or after complications related to the surgery."[5] Another factor is that weight-loss surgery has an average cost of $25,000 for each procedure. "The number of people eligible for the surgery is growing by an estimated 10 to 12 percent a year, and bariatric surgery can be profitable for hospitals and surgeons."[6]

I have four friends who have had gastric bypass surgery, and I have talked extensively with each of them. One common thread runs through every conversation: The emotional reasons for overeating in the first place must be dealt with and resolved for permanent success.

One of our First Place leaders in Kentucky has shared her story about her own weight-loss surgery. As you read it, pray and ask God what His will is for you.

My name is Sherry Benner. I am 35 years old. I am a mother of three children—ages 9, 7 and 3. I live in Elizabethtown, Kentucky, and am a registered nurse, a pastor's wife and a First Place leader.

I have been overweight since I was about 23 years old. I always had a tendency to gain weight, but because of being active, I didn't gain until I started nursing school, when I was 22. I sat and studied, stressed and ate for two solid years.

By the time I became pregnant for the first time, at the age of 24, I already weighed 196 pounds. I had difficult pregnancies, but I didn't overgain during them. I had my second baby 2½ years later and again had a difficult pregnancy. After my second son was born, I started keeping the weight on and feeling terrible all the time. I didn't sleep well, and I felt extremely self-conscious about my weight. We lived in the high-stress environment of the pastorate, and I used food a lot to deal with stress, disappointment, frustration, boredom and just about every other emotion I experienced. In between the births of my second son and my daughter, I had a miscarriage.

Finally, in January 2001, I had my daughter and weighed in at 246 pounds—my highest weight ever. In addition, the diabetes that I acquired from the pregnancy (I had insulin-dependent gestational diabetes with all the kids) did not leave. I had to be started on diabetic medication. Soon thereafter I was diagnosed with sleep apnea, which can be deadly. I was headed down a terrible road, and felt like I was at a crossroads—I had to change or I would die.

I had been a part of two First Place groups—both were wonderful. I loved the fellowship, friendships and Bible studies, and I did well with them. I lost weight each time. But this time felt different. I had two life-threatening conditions, plus high cholesterol and triglycerides and a family history of early heart disease and diabetic complications.

A friend from work was planning to have a gastric bypass and was talking about it at work. I felt like most people did: Gee, that is drastic and dangerous. Is she crazy? *But she just told me some websites to look into so that I could research it for myself. My husband, Todd, flipped out when he saw me looking into it; he didn't want anything to do with it. He was scared that I might die.*

Over several months, I came to know more about it and shared some things with Todd. I knew I would never do it without God's OK and Todd's. We were about to move, so I started to look into doctors in Louisville, close to where we would be living. I found the one I thought was a possibility, so Todd and I went to an informational meeting. We were both moved by what we heard. We were also impressed by the doctor and his strict requirements for his patients.

To make a long story short, I had gastric bypass surgery on February 24, 2002. I have lost 73 pounds. I don't have diabetes or sleep apnea anymore. My cholesterol is normal. I enjoy life and my family, and I no longer obsess over what I look like.

I am also a First Place leader. Some may say that I don't have any business being a leader since I lost my weight the easy way and didn't lean on God for success. However, anyone who knows anything about this surgery and this journey would know that it isn't the easy way at all. And I have leaned on God every step of the way. I have learned a new way of eating and drinking. A lot of my bad habits are gone. But a lot of them aren't. I still want to eat too much and I still crave things that aren't good for me. I still have head hunger, and I want to snack all the time. Surgery doesn't cure these things—and I knew it wouldn't. There are ways to sabotage yourself even after the surgery: ice cream, chips, soft drinks and so on. These things are eaten easily and can pack the pounds back on.

That is where First Place comes in. When a local group decided to start a First Place ministry, I was thrilled—I knew it would be wonderful to have back in my life. First Place is about more than losing weight; it is about putting Jesus first in our lives and being healthy—not just skinny.

I have had 10 to 15 stubborn pounds that I couldn't lose. I know that some people might think that I would be very happy just having 10 to 15 pounds to lose. I have worked really hard to get down to just 10 to 15 pounds. But what has kept me from losing them is my stubbornness and not putting God first.

Matthew 6:33, which says to "seek first his kingdom and his righteousness, and all these things will be given to you as well," is one of my favorite verses. God, through First Place, has really been dealing with those stubborn issues of mine. I am trusting God for those last pounds to come off, and they are finally coming off. What is more important, though, is what God is doing inside my spirit. I am learning to put Him first and everything else will be added (or removed!) from me. I am so grateful for First Place and am glad for my unique spot in the ministry.

Don't think that because you may have, or have had, weight-loss surgery, you don't need First Place—you couldn't be more wrong. If you don't deal with the attitudes and dependence on food, instead of the Lord, for your satisfaction, you will be in the same spot that you were before surgery.

If you are a leader, love and support those who have had or want to have weight-loss surgery. They have a place in First Place. We need to minister to all types of people, not just cookie cutter people, who want to lose weight. We know that the most important part of First Place deals with the spirit; and although weight-loss surgery isn't ever a first option, people who opt for this route still need our love, our support and our help to learn to put Christ in first place!

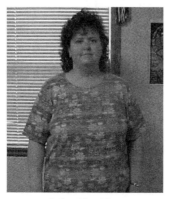
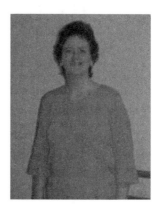

Before First Place   *Today*

MORE INFORMATION

For a more comprehensive look at the strengths and weaknesses of a wide array of popular diet plans, programs and strategies, please see the analysis from Colorado State professor and nutritionist Jennifer Anderson that follows this chapter.

Notes
1. *MYM Newsletter* (November 26, 2002).
2. "For Your Information," *Federal Trade Commission,* June 12, 2003. http://www.ftc.gov/opa/2003/06/2001cigrpt.htm (accessed August 23, 2004).
3. Richard Couey, *Nutrition For God's Temple,* (Lewiston, NY: Edwin Mellen Press, 1993), n.p.
4. M. Freudenheim, *New York Times* (August 29, 2003).
5. M. Ottey, *Seattle Times* (October 17, 2002).
6. M. Freudenheim, *New York Times* (August 29, 2003).

A Nutritionist Looks at Popular Diet Plans

by Jennifer Anderson, Ph.D., with L. Young

Quick Facts

Many diet products and programs offer a quick, short-term fix, but there is no "magic bullet" for weight loss. When investigating weight-loss products or programs, beware of high costs, pressure to buy special foods or pills, and fraudulent claims.

Diets

Approximately 50 million Americans go on a diet each year—yet only 5 percent keep the weight they lose off. Many trying to lose weight continually struggle to find an effective weight-loss method. Unfortunately, there is no "magic-bullet." The only proven way to lose weight and keep it off is by making permanent lifestyle changes. You must eat healthier, watch portion sizes and be active.

Even if you choose to use an over-the-counter weight-loss product or participate in a weight-loss program, the bottom line is that you still must eat fewer calories than you burn to lose weight. When selecting a weight-loss product or program, gather as much information as possible. . . .

EXAMPLES OF INEFFECTIVE DIET PRODUCTS

Diet patches. Removed from the market by FDA in the early 1990s because they were ineffective as a diet aid.

Magnet diet pills. Purportedly flush fat out of the body.

Certain bulk fillers (such as guar gum). May cause internal obstruction.

Electrical muscle stimulators. FDA may remove from market if promoted for weight loss.

Appetite-suppressing eyeglasses. Claim colored lenses project image on retina and decrease appetite.

Magic weight-loss earrings. Supposedly control hunger by stimulating acupuncture points.

WEIGHT-LOSS PRODUCTS

Diet-drink powdered formulas usually are mixed with a glass of milk and are substituted for one or more meals. Many users of these shakes report feeling constantly hungry and regain the lost weight when they give up the shakes. By relying on shakes, dieters follow artificial dieting methods and avoid learning how to work food into their lives.

Many prescription diet medicines have side effects and may not work for long-term weight loss. Over-the-counter pills containing the appetite suppressant PPA (phenylpropanolamine hydrochloride) can raise blood pressure. Over-the-counter pills containing ephedra may cause serious side effects, including dizziness, increased blood pressure or heart rate, chest pain, heart attack, stroke, seizure and even death. Currently, the Food and Drug Administration (FDA) is taking action to limit and/or ban the use of PPA and ephedra in over-the-counter medications and dietary supplements.

Example of a Nutritional Program[1]
Characteristics: Replaces two meals a day with . . . "shakes" and tablets.

Strengths: One meal per day of regular food advocated. Shakes generally include nonfat dry milk.

Weaknesses: Heavy reliance on . . . powders and tablets. Suggested rate of weight loss is too high (2½ to 7½ pounds/week).

Comments: Weight loss is never "fun and easy" as claimed. Reliance on a specific product does not teach healthy, lifelong eating habits.

Example of a Formula

Characteristics: Drink [sample] formula. Eat according to specified diet. Formula contains "antifat" weapon.

Weaknesses: Diet de-emphasized. Behavior modification lacking. Emphasis on speed of weight loss.

Comments: Formula probably contains an appetite suppressant.

Example of an Over-the-Counter Weight-Loss Product

Characteristics: Weight-loss program recommends two shakes/day (powder and milk), a snack and a complete dinner of 500 to 650 calories.

Strengths: Plan encourages regular exercise.

Weaknesses: Promotes use of brand-name frozen entrees and snack bars. Does not teach good eating habits.

Comments: Difficult to maintain weight loss once shakes are discontinued.

Second Example of an Over-the-Counter Weight-Loss Product

Characteristics: Weight loss program recommends three shakes/day (powder and skim milk), and a complete dinner of 500 to 650 calories.

Strengths: Low-fat, nutrient-rich foods are encouraged for dinner.

Weaknesses: Does not promote healthy eating habits.

Comments: Difficult to maintain weight loss once shakes are discontinued.

Diet Pills Containing PPA

Characteristics: Take capsule once or twice a day. Follow diet plan that comes with capsules. Pills suppress appetite, but weight loss occurs from following diet plan. Most brands have a diet plan enclosed. Many of these are good diets.

Weaknesses: Pills produce side effects that have not been adequately studied.

Comments: Weight loss comes from following the diet, not from taking the pills.

Diet Pills Containing Ephedra (also called Ma Huang)

Characteristics: Claims to promote weight loss. Take tablets daily. Recommended number of tablets varies depending on the product manufacturer.

Weaknesses: Pills can produce potentially life-threatening side effects. Side effects have not been adequately studied.

Comments: Ephedra is a central nervous system stimulant that suppresses appetite. Often combined with caffeine, which can increase risk for adverse side effects. Not proven safe or effective for weight loss.

Glucomannan Supplements

Characteristics: Follow 1,000-calorie per day diet and take two capsules before each meal. Claim that capsules reduce appetite and decrease food absorption.

Weaknesses: Claim weight loss of ½ to 1 pound/day. Sensational, nutritionally inaccurate presentation.

Comments: Glucomannans are naturally occurring food thickeners. Not yet proven safe or effective. Weight loss probably comes from following the diet.

Chitosan Supplements

Characteristics: Pills contain a dietary fiber derived from the shells of shellfish. Claim that taking the pills will reduce fat absorption, lower cholesterol and promote weight loss. Typical recommendations are to take 2-6 grams of chitosan per day, divided into doses of 1 gram with each meal.

Weaknesses: May cause gas, bloating and diarrhea. At high intakes, may interfere with absorption of fat-soluble vitamins.

Comments: Studies have shown weight loss occurs only when chitosan supplements are combined with a low-fat, reduced calorie diet.

Chromium Supplements

Characteristics: Claims that pills will lower blood sugar, reduce body fat, control hunger, reduce cholesterol and triglyceride levels, and increase muscle mass. Supplements are usually available as chromium salts, which help increase the absorption of chromium.

Weaknesses: One form of chromium, called chromium picolinate, may cause adverse side effects, including anemia, memory loss and DNA damage.

Comments: Roughly 50 percent of scientific studies have shown chromium has a beneficial effect, while the remaining studies have shown no effect.

St. John's Wort Supplements

Characteristics: Claims that supplementing with St. John's wort will suppress appetite and promote weight loss.

Weaknesses: Side effects may include gastrointestinal discomfort, tiredness, insomnia and mild allergic reactions.

Comments: According to the Food and Drug Administration, St. John's wort has not been proven safe or effective for weight loss. Not recommended for children, or for pregnant or breast-feeding women.

Green Tea Extract Supplements

Characteristics: Pills contain polyphenols, which are extracted from green tea and are thought to be strong antioxidants. May help lower cholesterol and triglycerides, and enhance weight loss.

Weaknesses: Extracts that also contain caffeine may lead to restlessness and/or insomnia.

Comments: More studies are still needed to determine if green tea extracts are beneficial for weight loss. Choose extracts that have a "standardized polyphenol content." People taking aspirin or blood-thinning medications should consult their doctor before taking green tea extracts, because green tea extracts may interfere with blood clotting.

Spirulina Supplements (Algae Tablets)

Characteristics: (1) Take tablets as an appetite suppressant before meals, or (2) replace evening meals with 6-10 spirulina tablets, or (3) in a modified fast, take only spirulina and drink juice for several days.

Strengths: Spirulina does contain essential nutrients and can be an acceptable food when used as part of a varied diet.

Weaknesses: Taken in large amounts on top of an adequate diet, spirulina could lead to toxic levels of certain nutrients. Does not teach sound eating habits.

Comments: Tablets are expensive.

Jennifer Anderson, Ph.D., is a Cooperative Extension food science and human nutrition specialist and professor at Colorado State University, Fort Collins, Colorado. L. Young is a former graduate student.

Note

1. The original report used specific product names. Those names have been deleted here, but the analysis of these examples remains valid and is most helpful in making wise weight-loss choices.

Part II

FIRST STEPS TO CHANGE

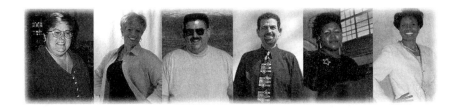

Chapter 3

NEW BEGINNINGS

*Reflect upon your present blessings, of which every man has many; not on your
past misfortunes, of which all men have some.*

CHARLES DICKENS

Perhaps when you were a child your family moved to a different town,
and you had to begin again at a new school and make new friends.
Maybe your parents got divorced and then remarried; you had to face the
trauma of your family splitting up and simultaneously adjust to a new
stepfather or stepmother. Possibly, due to a downturn in the economy,
you lost a job you had held for years. You were forced to find new
employment; maybe you had to switch to a new career.

Everyone will experience a point in time when he or she must start
anew; most of us have faced many such crossroads of change. Beginning
again is a very real part of life; but just because starting anew is inevitable
doesn't mean we like doing it. In fact, many of us fight change and resist
new beginnings. When it comes to losing weight, most of us have started over so many times that we simply cannot bear the thought of taking
that first step (or looking at that scale) one more time—but we must.
And it all starts with the first step.

STEPS TOWARD SUCCESS

Let's first focus on the importance of starting over. Beginning something (anything) again has the potential to take us from where we are to where we want to go, no matter the aspect of life that needs an adjustment.

Losing weight and keeping it off for a lifetime comes when we learn, not in our head but in our heart, that we can begin again anywhere, anytime. If we make an unhealthy choice at a meal, we don't need to wait until the next Monday to begin again. We can start anew with the next bite that goes into our mouth.

> Lucille had lost 42 pounds over a period of seven months. Even though she still needed to lose another 100 pounds, she was well on her way to victory. She had established a testimony of God's power and grace in her life—a testimony that was moving forward instead of standing still.

Success in losing weight and in every area of life comes by learning to begin again sooner rather than later. The hours, days, months and years will pass whether we begin again or wait, so we should think about where we will be two years from now if we choose to stay where we are today.

Caught by Surprise

At Christmas 2003, my husband, Johnny, was ill with a virus and unable to attend any of our family's celebrations. I stayed home with him on Christmas Eve while everyone else opened gifts together at our daughter Lisa's home. On Christmas Day, Johnny was somewhat better, so I had Christmas dinner with our family.

On the drive home, I stopped at a store to pick up something for Johnny to drink so he would not become dehydrated. I purchased three different flavors of Gatorade and decided to push the cart to my car. I opened the car doors with my automatic door opener, placed the heavy bottles on the floor by the back seat, shut the door, got in my car and drove away. When I arrived home and unloaded the car, I realized that I had left my purse in the shopping cart, which was in the busy parking lot. I called the store and asked them to check the carts for my purse, but it was gone.

Most women carry their lives in their purses, and I am no different. The next week I had to cancel credit cards, have my picture taken for a new driver's license, order new checks and purchase a new electronic address book. Almost three months later, I was still remembering additional items that were in that purse.

This story illustrates what beginning again can feel like. We're going through life when all of a sudden an event necessitates starting over. Sometimes we have known all along that our course needs to be altered. At other times, the event, announcement or circumstance creates or elevates a need to change.

Learning how and when to begin again can be the difference between success and failure.

Time to Change

What can spark change comes in many shapes and forms. For someone needing to lose weight, it might happen when we check the scale in the morning or look at the family reunion photos. It surely will grab our attention when a doctor tells us that our excess weight and sedentary lifestyle is going to lead to early death or a life lived in a wheelchair. When we find ourselves facing a future full of health problems, we know that we must begin again.

Starting over is a very real part of life. Frankly, learning how and when to begin again can be the difference between success and failure. Successful people not only comprehend this truth but they also set themselves free when they incorporate the practice of beginning again into their lifestyles. Simply put, those who accomplish their goals have learned how to begin again more quickly than those who miss the mark.

KEYS TO A FRESH START

I have discovered some keys that help me when I must begin again. Perhaps they will help you, too.

Acceptance of Circumstances

When it comes to my mom and my daughter Shari, I could choose to avoid reality; but the truth is that I will never again see either of them— not physically—here on Earth. I will, however, spend eternity with them because they both chose to follow Christ. Despite their physical absence, their lives and influence continue to play a role in my life and in the lives of their children and grandchildren—and I am certain that the influence will continue to flow for many generations to come. If I avoid the reality of their physical absence I will not see the beauty of their

> I'm not overweight. I'm just nine inches too short.
>
> —SHELLEY WINTERS

ongoing impact; seeing this impact is part of beginning again and moving on to live fully in the reality of new circumstances.

There comes a time in each of our lives when we must face the truth. Those of a younger generation call this a reality check. I call it seeing our circumstances as they really are rather than as we would like them to be. The particular circumstance can be anything with which we would rather not deal, such as losing a loved one, meeting a deadline or losing weight.

It really doesn't matter if our need to begin again is necessitated by our own bad choice, by someone else's bad choice or by circumstances. The simple truth is that until we accept our situation, we are not ready to begin again. Many of us live for months or years with feelings of anger, bitterness, hopelessness and fear, because we refuse to accept reality and start anew.

Some circumstances are easier to accept, others require more of God's grace. Recently, as I was writing in my prayer journal, I poured out my frustration and my own sin in regard to a particular set of circumstances in my life. As I resisted facing reality in this situation, I overate unhealthy foods and refused to exercise regularly. My prayer life was sporadic, because instead of taking my emotions to God and laying them at His feet, I carried them around, wallowing in self-pity. This behavior had characterized my life for two months—two months of self-defeating behavior that could have been two months of vibrant living, because I made the choice to stay where I was instead of deciding to begin again.

As I wrote about my distress and my pain, God came to me and began to speak quietly to my heart. I asked God to forgive me for my lack of belief, trust and obedience. As I opened my clenched fist, He began the process once again of changing my heart, and the Holy Spirit spoke truth to my soul.

The last truth God revealed to me during this time is that in the past He has repeatedly proved Himself to me. In January 2002, He wrote 90 devotional readings through me in eight days—just six weeks after Shari had died. In the fall of 2002, He wrote *Back on Track* through me as I believed, trusted and obeyed.

God only needs us to accept where we are, realizing that we have no power to do anything, in order for us to accomplish much. Does this sound confusing? It is a biblical principle that when we are weak we can be strong through Him (see 2 Cor. 12:9). God has the power and He wants us to draw on His power by being honest about the things He already knows about us, including our shortcomings.

Where are you right now? Does it seem as if life is about as bad as it can get? Tell God all about it; accept what you can't change and ask for forgiveness for your own contribution to where you find yourself at this moment. I don't know your circumstances but I imagine they aren't very different from circumstances many others have experienced throughout history. If you desperately need to lose excess pounds, then the first step is to accept reality. Where are you right now? Go ahead, take the first step and then watch God change your desires.

Willingness to Change

Once we accept reality, then we are ready to face the next hurdle: the challenge of actually making the needed changes so that we can get where we want to go. Having the willingness to change is probably the most difficult attitude to muster from within. Even though we might be miserable in our circumstances, the familiarity of our known misery always outweighs even the mere thought of changing. Change is uncomfortable. It means that we might have to do some things differently. It also means that we might have to stop doing some things that bring us pleasure and security.

Some years ago, our family was in a desperate situation. After months of acting like nothing was wrong, God clearly showed me through a caring friend the truth of my situation. Two weeks after accepting reality, our pastor, Dr. John Bisagno, preached a sermon on a person's will. I will never forget what he said that day. Our pastor said that God is a perfect gentleman who will never come in and forcibly change our will. He said that if we know that we are not willing to change then we can say this simple prayer: "Lord, I am not willing, but I am willing to be made willing." This prayer gives God permission to come in and do the work needed to change our stubborn wills.

After hearing that sermon, I was ready for God to take me to the next step necessary to bring about the changes I desired. As earnestly as I had ever sought God, I prayed that prayer. I was on the church staff and I didn't want anyone to know what a mess my life was in at that time, so I didn't go forward when the pastor called people to the altar at the close of the service that day. Nonetheless, at the end of the prayer, I begged God to not let the change hurt too much. I can honestly say that God was turned loose in my life that January morning in 1985 and He hasn't yet finished with all He has planned to do in and through my life.

I have sometimes thought about how far I have come with God. I remember how easily He straightened out our financial problems once we took our hands off of them. Twenty short years have whizzed by, and what a joyous ride it has been with God doing the driving! Even today when I contemplate a task I would rather not do, my heart is comforted with the same truth I learned 20 years ago. If I am not willing, God can make me willing—all I have to do is ask.

God had to get me to a desperate place to get my attention. How about you? Will you tell God how miserable you are and give Him permission to work on your will so that He can gently and lovingly teach you how to make the needed changes? You have my word that He will not stop until the job is done. Our part is to be willing to change.

THE THREE CS OF CHANGE

Along this wondrous ride, I have learned much, including some core principles about starting over. I call them the Three Cs of Change.

1. clarity
2. competence
3. continuous learning

Clarity
We can never make permanent changes in our lives unless we know exactly what changes need to be made. Zig Ziglar tells us that we need to be "a meaningful specific instead of a wandering generality."[1] Until we know exactly what we want, it is impossible to make a change in the right direction.

Let's review the steps. We need to

1. accept where we are.
2. become willing to change.

To achieve the task at hand, we must have clarity about what we need to do and how we are going to go about accomplishing it. If we need to clear our calendars to perform a certain task, then we must rearrange our schedules. Next, we have to actually do the things that we have identified.

In weight loss, clarity about what you want to accomplish is essential. How much weight do you want to lose? If you lose one to two pounds a week, how long will it take to reach your goal? How do you intend to accomplish this? Would it help to find an accountability partner or First

Place group to get the support you need? What changes must you make in your eating habits? Where and how are you going to exercise?

Just saying you need to lose weight or start exercising accomplishes nothing. You must learn how to actually act upon your good intentions. It has been said that the road to hell is paved with good intentions. Many of us live in our own personal hell on Earth because we never act on our good intentions.

I want to help you turn your good intentions into action. Please, take out a piece of paper and a pen or pencil. Write the numbers 1 to 10 on the paper. Now, in the first person voice, write ten things that you would like to change or see happen in your life 12 months from now. For example, one year from now these things will be true about the way I live:

1. I walk three miles, five days a week.
2. I do not eat fried foods or desserts.
3. I have memorized 52 verses of Scripture.
4. I respond in love to my spouse.
5. I do not scream at my children.
6. I am the best employee I can be.
7. I spend quality time with God every day.
8. I make it a point to encourage someone daily.
9. I manage my time.
10. I manage my finances.

Your list will be different from mine and you might be overwhelmed when you look at ten items that now seem impossible. Good! We all have to start over some time, some place. Now is a good time. Your assignment is to pick the one thing from this list of ten items that will help you the most and then work on it every day for the next year. When you do this, you will find that many of the other changes you desire will happen as by-products of your faithfulness to work on just one thing.

Clarity brings the knowledge of what we want and what we need to do to get it.

Competence

In the fall of 1984, I attended a women's retreat in Austin, Texas, and heard Patsy Clairmont teach about dreams. After telling us that only God places dreams into our hearts, Patsy asked us to think about something we would absolutely love to do and to write about that dream in a notebook. Patsy shared that she had always dreamed of being able to play the piano, but after finally being able to buy a piano in adulthood and taking piano lessons, she realized that she didn't want to do the hard work needed to become an accomplished pianist. Hearing her words that day, I realized that I had spent the last 25 years raising children and had never given a conscious thought to anything I might want to do. In my notebook, I wrote down that I was dreaming of doing what Patsy Clairmont was doing that day: talking and laughing with women who wanted to hear what she had to say. Bear in mind, I had never spoken publicly in my life. Nonetheless, I promised God that if He wanted to fulfill my newfound dream then I would promise to never say no to any offer to speak.

Immediately, I began to receive invitations. I was amazed when a number of Sunday school teachers asked me to speak to their classes. After giving a few devotional talks, I realized that public speaking was something I desired to do and I took steps to improve my skills. In 1985, I attended a three-day seminar called CLASS (Christian Leaders, Authors and Speakers Seminar) taught by Florence Littauer and learned the foundations of public speaking, such as creating an outline and how to gather subject matter by always being alert to situations around me. Over the next few years, God provided opportunities for me to become competent enough in my speaking skills so that He could expand my horizons and fulfill my dream.

By 1987, I was at a point that when offered the job of leading the First Place program, I felt competent enough to accept the challenge. For many people, public speaking is second only to death as their greatest fear, but God has taught me that any dream He places in my heart can come to reality if I am willing to take the time to become competent.

Losing weight and developing physical fitness is not much different from learning to speak in public. We must first learn how to do it and then we must practice until we become proficient. When we practice good habits, we become what we practice. When we practice bad habits, we digress. The only way we are ever going to lose weight and keep it off is to permanently change our lifestyle.

Dieting simply does not work. A diet is something we go on while we continually think about when we will be done with it. A lifestyle is part of who we are: body, soul, mind and spirit. Only with a permanent lifestyle change can we hope to win the battle to lose weight and keep it off forever.

Only with a permanent lifestyle change can we hope to win the battle to lose weight and keep it off forever.

This is the reason I love the First Place program. The program focuses on the total person, not just the physical aspect. Even though I have failed many times, through 24 years of practicing the First Place principles, I have learned that they work. The more competent I become in consistently eating healthy foods and exercising regularly, the more I am assured of a healthy weight and a fit body. As I consistently practice the spiritual disciplines found in First Place (Scripture reading, Scripture memory, prayer and Bible study) I find that my life becomes balanced spiritually. As I refuse to believe the lies of the enemy and focus on God's truth, my life becomes emotionally balanced. As I mentally contemplate what God desires for me to do, and then set out to actually do it, my mind comes into balance.

I recognize that most people come to a weight loss program to lose weight. But to really succeed, these four areas—the physical, the spiritual, the emotional and the mental—must all be in balance. Only then can we live a healthy, happy lifestyle. This is not easy, but it is possible. Our job is to become competent in changing our lifestyle from that of a wandering generality to that of a meaningful specific.

Continuous Learning

After we become clear about what we want, we must become competent to do the necessary work to accomplish our goals. Why is this not enough? Because the first two Cs of clarity and competence focus on self and the last C of continuous learning helps us focus on others. This is where we will find our ultimate joy in life.

I do not want to stop learning—ever. For this reason, I read and listen all the time. Each day I spend two hours commuting. I use the time to listen to Christian messages or Christian music. When on an airplane, I read books and magazines so that I can learn more and share what I have learned with others. I teach a First Place class every Tuesday at noon so that I can keep my finger on the pulse of the program. By leading others and seeing the changes that take place as they give Christ first place in their lives, I am motivated and inspired to continue doing what I do.

Some observers might think that my ministry in life is to direct First Place. Although I dearly love First Place, I love the people in the program more than the program itself. I will eventually retire from directing the First Place program, but I will never retire from loving the people in the program. As I continue to learn about God and about His people, He will continue to use me in the ministry He has given me. My job may come to an end, but my God-given ministry will not end until the day God calls me home. For this reason, I personally do not believe in "retirement."

One of my heroes is Marge Caldwell, a 90-year-old member of my church. I first came to know Marge when I was 9. She was one of my teachers, and her life has continued to teach me since that time. I have watched Marge as cancer took away her only daughter. I have watched her as she has endured physical trials. Marge is the most amazing woman, and she most certainly is the kind of woman I want to be when I am her age. Marge still counsels women as a part-time member of our church staff and she serves on our pastor search committee. She is always on the go and still teaches. Not long ago, I received an invitation to attend a Christian Business Women's luncheon. You guessed it; Marge was the keynote speaker.

Continuous learning is vital to permanent change. While we learn, God can continue to use us mightily—no matter our age.

After we lose the weight we want to lose and after we become physically fit, the key to permanent change is giving back to others the gift God has given to us. If you choose to "tell another hungry beggar where to find the bread"[2] you will continue to be fed yourself.

THE BIG STEP

The final and most important aspect of beginning again is to call on God for the help we need. I have placed this step last after *accepting where we are* and *being willing to change* because calling on God is usually the last thing we do.

Most people do exactly what I did after losing my purse. They think, brood and ruminate on their condition for months, maybe years, before they do the one thing that will help their situation, and that is to pray.

When my children were small, I delighted in meeting their needs. I knew their obvious requirements of food, clothing, shelter and love, so I provided those for them. When my children were young, the real satisfaction came when they approached me and asked for my help when something was troubling them. I still like to provide love and counsel to my children when they ask, but I rarely give counsel when they don't seek it.

It is the same with our heavenly Father. God delights in meeting our needs, but He wants us to ask for His help when anything troubles us or when we have lost our way. He longs to give us the desires of our hearts, if we will only ask.

I have another assignment for you. Sit down and write a letter to God. Tell Him about the troubles in your life. Yes, He already knows the details, but He desperately wants to hear them from you because He wants to have a close, loving relationship with you, His child. Tell Him about all of the times that you have tried to lose weight. Tell Him about your family and financial problems. After you have poured out your heart to God, ask for His help to make the changes you so desperately want and need.

> Call to me and I will answer you and tell you great and unsearchable things you do not know.
>
> —JEREMIAH 33:3

When we pray, our God instantly springs into action to provide answers. This is a miracle that I don't begin to understand but I joyfully accept. God knows how we are, and the Bible is full of stories of men and women just like you and me. That's what I love about the Bible. God didn't sugarcoat the stories about the people He used mightily. The Bible tells us the bad things as well as the good things these people said and did. It records how God helped them every time they asked for His help. This holy book is still living and active today. As we read and study it, the truths therein become our guidebook for living. Prayer, though, is the secret ingredient for permanent change.

Jesus modeled the practice of prayer as He lived on Earth. He constantly prayed to His Father for wisdom and guidance. Why? Because Jesus was confined to a fleshly body for the 33 years He lived on Earth. His body faced all of the temptations and desires we face every day, but the Bible records that Jesus lived a sinless life. He was able to do so because He never did or said anything unless His Father told Him to do or say it. Read the Bible and see for yourself. Repeatedly in the four Gospels (Matthew, Mark, Luke and John) Jesus refers to spending time with God. In fact, the New Testament reveals that often Jesus prayed early in the morning. It also records that He sent the disciples away so that He could spend time talking with Father God. If Jesus needed to pray, how much more important is it for us to pray?

When we call on God for help, we receive His wisdom instead of our own. He will guide our day and our thoughts.

The Lord saw how great man's wickedness on the earth had become, and that every inclination of the thoughts of his heart was only evil all the time (Gen. 6:5).

If the Bible is true—and I believe that it is—and if Jesus set an example for us to follow, then we need to ask God to direct our thoughts and our actions each day. Our lives stay balanced when God guides the decisions we make and the steps we take. God has never failed to help me when I ask for His help. I am confident the same will be true for you as you practice prayer.

> One of my favorite verses is Isaiah 30:21: "Whether you turn to the right or to the left, your ears will hear a voice behind you saying, 'This is the way, walk in it.'"

Losing weight and keeping it off is a huge problem for many people today. I am thrilled to tell you that your desire to take off your excess pounds is no problem at all for God. He is ready and waiting to help if you will just call out to Him. He will send people into your life to teach you but even better than that, He Himself will guide you into all truth.

Notes

1. Zig Ziglar, quoted at *Motivational-Depot.com*. http://www.motivationaldepot.com/speakers/authors (accessed on October 11, 2004).
2. D. T. Niles, quoted in *Simpson's Contemporary Quotations*, compiled by James B. Simpson (New York: Houghton Mifflin Company, 1988), n.p.

SHEILA ROBBINS

E-Newsletter Editor
Houston, Texas

I have been a part of the First Place program since September 1985—as a member, leader, First Place staff member and sometimes as a spokesperson. I went from 320 pounds to 163 pounds and kept those pounds off for more than 12 years.

However, for the next six years I began a roller-coaster ride. I struggled with maintaining my weight and by 2003, I had gained back almost 50 pounds. I periodically joined First Place classes, but never seemed to lose weight. I knew what I needed to do, but I could not motivate myself to stay on track.

After sharing my struggles with Carole Lewis and other First Place members, Carole sent me her book *Back on Track*. She handwrote inside, "I pray this book blesses you!" Carole also inscribed a reference to Romans 15:13: "May the God of hope fill you with all joy and peace as you trust in him, so that you may overflow with hope by the power of the Holy Spirit." As I looked for the verse in my Bible, I began to pray for God to intervene in my life. I knew I had lost hope of staying healthy, even after 12 years of maintaining my weight. I knew what needed to be done: to regain any hope, I had to place my eyes back on the Lord and recommit myself to Him.

After reading *Back on Track*, I had a renewed spirit. Every chapter spoke to me, describing my "battle with my bulges." I realized that I had been trying to live without joy and peace. The Holy Spirit showed me how my own worries, circumstances and other people's actions had worn me down and robbed me of my joy in Christ. Now, when I come face-to-face with these joy killers, I remember Romans 15:13. My God of hope has again filled me with joy and peace, as I trust Him daily. As I do

His will, I trust in Him to get healthy.

As of the writing of this book, I have lost 25.5 pounds. As I continue to desire His will, I receive His joy. My Lord again has first place in my life.

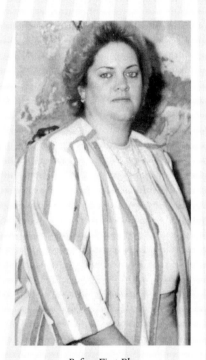

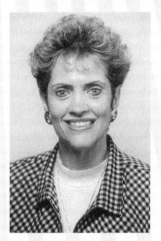

Today

Before First Place

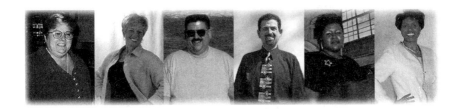

BAROMETERS OF HEALTHY WEIGHT

All successful people have a goal. No one can get anywhere unless he knows where he wants to go and what he wants to be or do.

NORMAN VINCENT PEALE

How do you go about deciding that you need to lose weight and how much you need to lose? Do you look in the mirror? Depend on the bathroom scale? Only worry when the doctor tells you that your health is in serious jeopardy? While these barometers indeed offer hints about your physical fitness, or lack thereof, you can get a better grasp on your current status. Before you begin to lose weight in earnest, it helps to know the condition of your body. This knowledge will help determine the personal weight-loss and health goals you set for yourself.

GROWING LARGER

If you have gotten this far in this book, it is likely that you are one of the oversized Americans who wants to slim down and become better fit. Let's start with a basic self-examination.

- Has your weight been increasing steadily over the last several years?
- What changes in your life and lifestyle may be contributing to your weight gain?

These certainly are not the only indicators; however, if you answered yes to the first question, then you probably have already concluded that you need to lose weight. That brings us to the next question: What changes in your life and lifestyle may be contributing to your weight gain? There may be more factors, but start by listing three of them here:

1.

2.

3.

Many experts attribute increasing levels of obesity to the demands of modern living and the lifestyles we choose to live. Longer work hours and more time spent in our cars leave less time for physical activity and make healthy eating more difficult. Television remote controls, computers, self-propelled lawnmowers and fast-food drive-through windows (with the possible lure of a free quesadilla) have become part of everyday life. While modern technology is good, it decreases opportunities for physical activity at home and at work. Combined with easy access to a variety of high-calorie, high-fat and good-tasting food, modern lifestyles make it very difficult to achieve and maintain a healthy weight.

While weight gain results from an imbalance between calorie intake and energy expenditure, weight regulation is actually a complex process in which physical, hormonal, environmental, genetic, emotional and social issues can influence metabolism, appetite, body composition, activity levels and lifestyle choices.

The popular view is that obesity is an issue of willpower and choice; moreover, fad diets that place the blame on certain foods or one specific cause are too simplistic and can be misleading.

ACHIEVING A HEALTHY WEIGHT

As noted in chapter 1, people with poor dietary habits and physical inactivity not only risk becoming obese, they also endanger their health and their lives. Major problems faced by overweight people can include coronary heart disease, diabetes, cancer, gallbladder disease, stroke, high blood pressure, arthritis and infertility.

The biggest danger, however, is death. Each year, more than 300,000 overweight or obese Americans die. In fact, problems caused by poor dietary habits and physical inactivity are the second leading cause of preventable death in the United States.

Scientific evidence now shows that a weight loss of just 5 to 10 percent can significantly reduce—and even reverse—the negative health effects associated with being overweight or obese. Moderate weight loss is also associated with an improved quality of life. With such raw evidence, many experts are abandoning the concept of ideal weight in favor of healthier weight.

What are your health risks? Answer the following questions honestly:

- Do you have any have any obesity-related diseases or health risks? If you don't know your risk factors, visit your doctor for a checkup.
- Because some diseases and risk factors don't develop until later in life, it's important to look at what problems run in your family. Do any obesity-related diseases or health risks run in your family?
- Do you believe that losing weight will help lower your risk factors?

- Are you ready to commit to losing 10 percent of your current weight (if you're overweight) to improve your health?
- Multiply your current body weight by .9 to determine your healthier weight.
- Are you willing to make the lifestyle changes necessary to achieve and maintain your healthier weight, even if you can't achieve your ideal weight?

THE BODY-MASS INDEX

The worksheet below will help you set goals and track your progress. Experts now use Body-Mass Index (BMI) to help determine if a person's weight is putting his or her health at risk. A healthy weight is not about physical appearance or a number on the scale. In most people, BMI provides an accurate reflection of body composition and health risks. Some people who are very muscular and fit can have a high BMI yet be very lean and healthy.

Another important measure in addition to BMI is waist circumference. Men with a waist circumference greater than 40 inches and women

HOW TO CALCULATE YOUR BMI

Multiply your current weight in pounds by 703.
Weight _____ x 703 = (a)

Divide the result (a) by your height in inches.
(a) _____ ÷ height _____ = (b) _____

Divide the result (b) by your height in inches.
(b) _____ ÷ height _____ = BMI

Understanding Your BMI

< 20	Weight loss not indicated
20 to 25	This is your healthy weight range
26 to 30	Increasing health risk
> 30	Obesity and high health risk
> 40	Very high health risk

with one greater than 35 inches are particularly high risk for weight-related diseases, such as heart disease and diabetes. Regardless of a person's weight or BMI, a high waist measurement indicates that there is excess fat in the abdomen, which leads to increased health risks.

To measure your waist circumference, take a measurement with a tape measure placed in the one-inch space located just below your bottom rib and above the top of your hipbone (for most people this is about the level of the navel).

SETTING GOALS

One of the best things you can do for your overall health is to prevent any further weight gain. In fact, studies show that following a healthy lifestyle of good nutrition and regular physical activity is more important to your overall health and well-being than what you weigh. Committing yourself to a healthy lifestyle and maintaining your present weight are important, and both are worthwhile goals.

Many people have unrealistic expectations about their bodies and ideal body weight. We live in a society that values a lean and fit body, but a healthy weight is not necessarily the popular ideal. More important than having a lean and fit body are living a healthy lifestyle and maintaining a weight that's associated with good health and abundant living. A healthy weight considers who you are emotionally, spiritually, intellectually, physically and socially. Your goal should be to follow a lifestyle that's in balance with God's overall desire for your life. In later chapters I go into greater detail about these all-important factors.

Go ahead and start thinking about some goals, even if you do not know how to achieve them right now. How many total pounds would

---

A healthy weight considers who you are emotionally, spiritually, intellectually, physically and socially.

---

you like to lose? How many do you think you can lose in a week? What eating habits will you need to change? What lifestyle factors will you need to alter? In First Place, individuals set goals with the help of a group. Most of you reading this book will not have a group, so I suggest you find an individual—a friend, relative, coworker or someone else whom you trust. This person can be a great help to you as you start out and as you set realistic goals.

Also, seek God's advice. He may very well be the One prompting you to start a weight-loss plan. He certainly wants you to be healthy. You can say a prayer something like the following one:

> *Dear Lord, I know that I have a lot of weight to lose, and this fact sometimes overwhelms me. I am asking for Your help to lose the first 10 percent of the total amount of weight I need to lose. Please help me do my part to make wise food choices and to begin exercising, and then help me trust You for the weight-loss results. In Jesus' name I pray. Amen.*

JENN KROGH

Kewaunee, Wisconsin

There are three stages to my story, and each one represents a picture of being lost, being found, moving forward and becoming the woman God created me to be.

In 1986, I was the heaviest I had ever been in my life, and I believe that the weight was an outward physical display of the amount of bondage, pain and stress I was carrying. In 1988, I accepted Christ's invitation to be my Savior, and God began an inward transformation of me. Five years later, it was time to begin to shed the physical layers that were weighing me down. I joined another Christian weight-loss program and lost 87 pounds. I even led weight-loss groups. However, I did not have the accountability that I needed. I was unable to lose as much weight as I wanted to lose before that Christian program shut its doors.

I didn't give up; I just did not know where to turn until early in the fall of 2001, when I came in contact with First Place. I have not been the same since. We started a First Place group here in Kewaunee, Wisconsin. Throughout all of my years of leading weight-loss groups prior to First Place, there was wonderful Christian fellowship and support and some weight loss, but I have never seen such a truly Spirit-inspired program as First Place. I now have the wonderful privilege of seeing lives changed. Members have lost weight and improved their physical health, but even more important, they have grown spiritually and emotionally. They have been healed, and they continually have their minds renewed by God.

I reached my goal weight on December 17, 2001. It has been a journey and a process that continues. For various reasons, including age and the use of medications, I still struggle to maintain my weight. But I am committed to First Place, and I know that I can succeed. God never fails and neither will you when you apply the truth and use the tools provided in First Place.

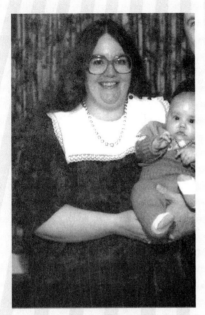
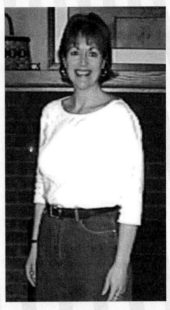

Before First Place   *Today*

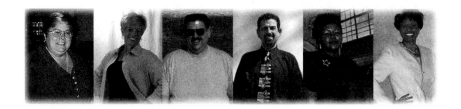

C h a p t e r 5

THE PHYSICAL CONNECTION

Habits are funny things. What's funny, or rather tragic, is that bad habits are so predictable and avoidable. Despite this, there are people by the millions who insist on acquiring habits that are bad, expensive, and create problems. The habit they weren't going to get, got them!

ZIG ZIGLAR

When our veterinarian told my husband, Johnny, that our dog, Meathead, was too heavy and that disability, or an early death, could be the consequence if we did not help him lose weight, Johnny sprang into action. He started the process by weaning Meathead from some bad habits.

The habit of taking Meathead to a local café each morning had to stop. Why? The cook always gave Meathead a free sausage and biscuit. All wieners and cheese were now banished from Meathead's life. Johnny loves Meathead so much that he began carefully measuring Meathead's (now dry) dog food and discontinued feeding the dog unhealthy snacks.

No more Shake's frozen custard! This franchise gives a free cup to any pet riding in the car.

How many times does our personal physician have to tell us to lose weight before we figure out how to do it? It usually takes much more than a warning from our doctor to propel us to lose weight and start exercising. For literally millions of Americans, changes are not begun until after we have had a stroke or a heart bypass surgery. Too many wait until diabetes has already taken its toll on our bodies through the loss of eyesight or a limb.

The physical connection includes three links: food, exercise and accountability.

FOOD

The First Place food plan is flexible, easy to learn, and men and women all over the world are losing weight the First Place way. For those who are unable or for whatever reason choose not to join a First Place class, we have included a 30-day First Place eating plan at the back of this book. This plan can be used indefinitely until you reach your target weight. The 30-day food plan is flexible, because you can choose any one of the 30 suggested breakfasts, lunches or dinners. The plan is easy, because meals are chosen from foods available at home to foods from a fast food restaurant, and every meal, in each category, has the same number of calories.

Many lunch and dinner meals include easy recipes that your family will enjoy, without feeling deprived. Our First Place chef, Scott Wilson, has chosen recipes, low in fat and sugar, that are easy to make, nourishing and taste good.

Being able to mix and match meals takes the complexity out of losing weight. The beauty of this 30-day plan is that no matter which breakfast, lunch or dinner you choose, your daily calories will total 1,400. An added benefit is that this 30-day plan follows the USDA guidelines for healthy eating.

First Place recommends that no one lose more than two pounds per week. If after the first three weeks you are losing more than two pounds weekly, begin eating a double portion at one of the meals and know that you are still eating healthfully. The goal is to eat enough calories to lose no more than two pounds each week.

EXERCISE

Exercise is a vital link to permanent weight loss for two reasons. The first reason to exercise is that regular exercise turns our bodies into efficient calorie-burning machines. It doesn't matter if you can barely walk today. If you will begin barely walking, God will reward your efforts by helping you do a little more each day. Joe Ann Winkler's testimony reveals God's power to work when we ask for His help. (Read more about Joe Ann Winkler in her testimonial, which follows this chapter.)

Exercise is a vital link to permanent weight loss.

The second reason to develop a lifestyle that includes exercise is to keep from regaining the weight after we lose it. In First Place, when we reach our permanent weight-loss goal, we begin adding back calories so that we do not continue to lose weight. Adding calories and stopping our exercise is a recipe for weight gain.

How much exercise do I need?
A person who is in poor physical condition needs to exercise five days each week to begin developing physical fitness. After we gain physical fit-

ness, it is good to never go longer than 48 hours without exercise.

How hard do I need to exercise?

In the beginning, do what you can. Walking is a wonderful way to begin your exercise program. At first, you may only be able to make it down the street and back before reaching your target heart range and needing to stop. The goal is to eventually work up to walking three miles, four to five days a week.

First Place and Body and Soul, a Christian aerobics program, partnered to develop two DVDs for use in establishing a lifestyle of fitness. These DVDs cover the three important components of fitness: aerobic capacity, flexibility and strength training.

For more information on becoming physically fit, parts 3 and 4 in this book answer the most frequently asked questions about food and exercise.

ACCOUNTABILITY

Accountability is the link between desire and discipline. For most of us, the journey to lose weight and become physically fit is made easier when we are joined by others. First Place has been successful in helping men and women reach their goal to lose weight and keep it off because accountability is built into every facet of the program.

1. We attend a small group meeting once a week for 13 weeks. As the group bonds, we are able to be accountable to each other.
2. We encourage one other person in our group each week with a card, phone call or e-mail. This simple accountability tool helps us learn to focus more on others than on ourselves.
3. In class we discuss the Bible study that we studied during the previous week. Knowing that we will talk about the study helps us stay accountable to actually do the study at home.

4. We say our weekly memory verse when we step on the scale to weigh each week. The accountability of actually saying the verse helps us to memorize it, and the verse also takes the focus off of weighing.

5. The accountability of weighing each week helps us remember to eat healthy foods and to exercise so that we can show a weight loss instead of a gain.

6. We check off how we are doing in all the areas of the program on our Commitment Record and turn it in to our leader. This is another area of accountability that is vital to our overall success in developing a balanced lifestyle.

Knowing about the value of accountability won't help us unless we learn to embrace accountability as a friend. Over the last 20 years, accountability has become the link that keeps my life balanced in all areas. To ensure that I exercise regularly, I meet a friend to walk. As we walk each day, we say our Scripture memory verses together. Leading a First Place class each week helps me stay accountable to my class members. Routines help to develop accountability. Showing up for work five days a week, on time, ensures that I continue to receive my paycheck. The accountability is established because I want to keep being paid for the job I do. This same principle holds true in any area where we need balance. Adding the link of accountability will be the added impetus to get us off dead center and moving toward wholeness.

JOE ANN WINKLER

Overland Park, Kansas

I have had MS (multiple sclerosis) since 1950, when I was 16 years old. Doctors originally diagnosed my condition as polio. I did not learn that it was MS until two decades later. From the time I was 16 to this day I have only been able to walk short distances.

In 1971, I had double pneumonia and was in critical condition for three weeks. When the medical staff at the hospital attempted to have me walk, I couldn't. I was fitted in a full leg brace on my right leg and a half brace on my left leg. I used a wheelchair from that time on. In 1972, I went into the hospital for a hernia repair. The doctors called in a specialist, and the hospital staff did a number of tests, including a spinal tap. That is when they determined that I actually suffered from MS and not polio. Because of my medical condition and the resulting sedentary lifestyle, I became overweight.

I joined First Place in 1993 and lost 100 pounds. Due to the steroids I had to take for the MS, I gained most of it back over the years. During that time I also became a First Place group and area leader.

In July 2003, I attended a leadership meeting in Houston, Texas. While there, I purchased a copy of Carole Lewis's book, *Back on Track*. A week or so after I returned home I sat down to read the book and I was fully inspired. I bought a bracelet that had the words "believe," "trust" and "obey" inscribed on it. I wanted to believe I could lose weight again, trust God to help me and obey His directions, but I could not exercise enough to get the results I wanted. I thought about the three words on my bracelet, and Philippians 4:13 immediately came to mind: "I can do everything through him who gives me strength."

Could God override my MS and give me the ability to walk for exercise? I decided to trust Him and see if I could actually walk more than a few steps. I wasn't being obedient by sitting around thinking about

walking. I had to act on my faith. I started out with just a few steps outdoors and kept going a little farther each day. I prayed to be able to walk
just a mile. *If I could do that, I would be so happy*, I thought. God gave me
that mile!

One day it was raining and I was very disappointed that I could not
walk outdoors. My husband, Jack, said he would take me to the mall so
that I could walk indoors, out of the rain. I walked at a snail's pace,
because I still had a fear of falling. Everyone passed me, so I decided to
use this time to pray—that was the start of my prayer walking. I know
now that it was not me walking, but Christ walking through me.
Without Christ I am nothing.

I began to walk a little farther each day, and that gave me more
prayer time for more people. Before long I was walking two miles.
People, as they passed me, commented on how much better I was walking. I was still slow. One day Jack told me that he thought I could pass a
particular elderly man who was walking with a cane. I just wanted to be
able to pass one person, so passing the elderly man became my goal.
Finally, I made it past him. It didn't matter that he was probably 80 years
old and had trouble walking, too. Isn't it curious how sometimes we
have such foolish little ideas?

My MS has not improved much. Doctors no longer prescribe the
medicine that helped me the most, and the new medicine does me harm
instead of good, so the doctor took me off of it. God has been good to
me, and the progression of MS has been very slow.

God has answered so many of my prayers while I have been letting
Him walk through me, and I love the times I can spend talking to my
heavenly Father. It doesn't matter what we are talking about—I just love
being in His presence.

I now walk three miles every morning. I kept track of my mileage,
and I hope that I will soon pass the 500-mile mark. One more thing: God
has blessed me with a 77-pound weight loss during nine months. What
a great God!

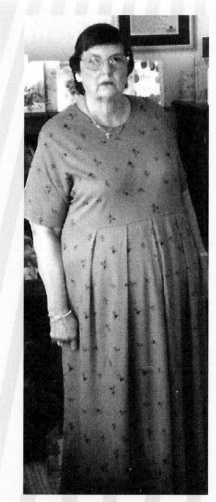

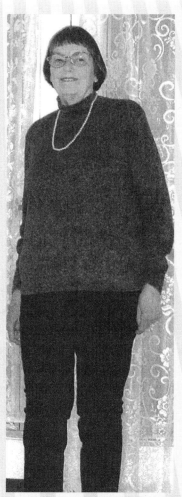

Before First Place   *Today*

Part III

THE FOOD CONNECTION

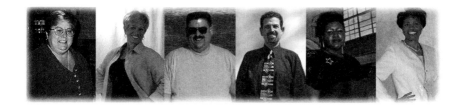

Chapter 6

THE NEW FOOD GUIDE PYRAMID

To stem the obesity epidemic, most Americans need to reduce the amount of calories they consume. When it comes to weight control, calories do count—not the proportions of carbohydrate, fat and protein in the diet.

FEDERAL ADVISORY PANEL

Most major health and nutrition organizations adopted the Food Guide Pyramid when it was introduced in 1992. Medical professionals, nutritionists and educators like the Pyramid because it offers a visual and practical way to put healthy nutrition into practice. The Pyramid, developed by the United States Department of Agriculture, divides all foods into five groups based on their nutritional similarities and the number of servings needed in a healthy diet. It includes an additional category for fats, oils and sweets and advises that these should be eaten sparingly.

The Food Guide Pyramid shows how each food group supplies some, but not all, of the nutrients that we need. No one food or food group is more important than another; we need them all for nutritional health. The Food Guide Pyramid recommends that we eat a variety of foods from each group and that we stick with the recommended number of servings to achieve our goals for healthy weight and good health.

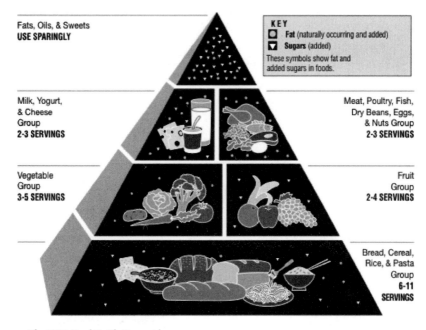

The 1992 Food Guide Pyramid

While the 1992 Food Guide is most helpful, it doesn't tell us what a serving size should look like. Since the beginning of the First Place program in 1981, we have taught our members about serving sizes. Correct serving sizes are the key to losing weight and keeping it off.

EXPANDED RECOMMENDATIONS

The USDA has developed a new Food Guide Pyramid and has scheduled to release it in 2005 (after the publication date of this book). At this writing, we don't yet know exactly what it will look like, but we do know that some of the recommendations are exciting; the guide will now inform the American people not only what to eat but how much to consume from each group.

The new program will have a new name: the Food Guide Pyramid/Food Guidance System. Here are some of the tools that the USDA will develop as the core of this new system:

- A graphic that serves as a visual representation of the overall food guidance system
- Clear, concise nutrition messages that teach consumers how to make healthier choices
- Tools that assist consumers in establishing healthier eating patterns and improve overall health
- Interactive tools that allow consumers to personalize the guidance for their specific needs[1]

One major change in the new Food Guide Pyramid is its intent to give individualized guidance instead of generalized information. With so many people needing to lose weight, one set of guidelines clearly will not work for everyone. This, again, is a tenet that has been taught in First Place for years. Here are some of the expected USDA guidelines:

- To improve their food choices, individuals need to have access to information specific to their own energy and nutrient needs, based on their age, sex, and physical activity level.
- Generalized messages provide less specific information—intended for all individuals—such as the range of 6 to 11 daily servings from the grains group. This information was misunderstood by some to mean they could choose anywhere within that range.
- Individualized guidance will identify that individuals of a certain age, sex, and activity level could have, for example, 6 ounce equivalents of grains (e.g., 6 slices of bread or [6] ounces of cereal) per day, while younger, more active individuals might have 8 ounce equivalents.[2]

The USDA assembled a panel to make recommendations for changes in the Food Guide Pyramid. While we do not yet know exactly how many of the recommendations will eventually be adopted, some of the conclusions are good news. Paralleling a basic principle First Place has taught since 1981, the committee wrote, "The healthiest way to reduce calorie intake is to reduce one's intake of added sugars, solid fat and alcohol—they all provide calories, but they do not provide essential nutrients."[3]

One major change recommended by the panel is breaking down vegetables into five categories, including dark greens and starchy ones. There are also some specific guidelines on what vegetables to eat, including the portion size:

- Three cups weekly of dark-green vegetables, such as broccoli or spinach
- Two cups of orange vegetables, including carrots and squash
- Three cups of legumes such as lentils and chickpeas
- Six cups of starchy vegetables such as potatoes, corn and green peas
- Seven cups of other vegetables, including tomatoes, onions and lettuce[4]

Eating fish—because it contains omega-three fatty acids—is high on the list of the panel's recommendations. Two servings—about eight ounces—per week would lower the risk of coronary heart disease, the panel suggests.

Other advice in the proposed guidelines includes the following:

- **Select** healthy carbohydrates, including whole-grain foods like whole-wheat bread, brown rice, whole-wheat pasta and oatmeal.
- **Choose** healthy fats. Oils high in poly- and monounsaturated fats such as olive, canola, corn and peanut are the best for your heart.
- **Pick** healthy sources of protein that are low in saturated fat, including nuts, legumes, fish, poultry and eggs, eaten in moderation.
- **Eat** plenty of fruits and vegetables. If you use canned products, look for "low-sodium" or "no salt added" on the label.[5]

How much dairy product Americans consume will shift if the panel's recommendations are adopted. Now everyone but small children is advised to consume two to three servings a day. That will be increased to a full three servings for adults.

The 1992 Food Guide Pyramid suggests people moderate the amount of sugar consumed. The new guidelines could use verbiage something like, "Choose your carbohydrates wisely," and may allow for a certain number of discretionary calories, about 10 percent of a person's daily diet.[6]

The new food pyramid guide could look something like the graphic below, although we will not know for certain until the FDA makes its changes official.

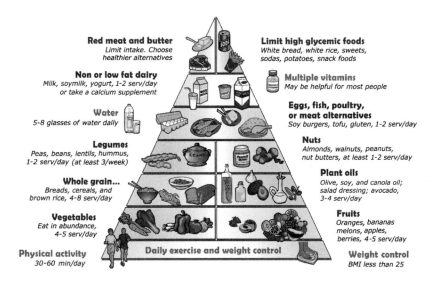

What the new Food Guide Pyramid may look like.
New Food Pyramid design developed by Wellsource, Inc. © 2004. Used by permission.

Cutting through the maze of new recommendations from the USDA, we find that the new federal guidelines substantially offer much of the same information that First Place has been teaching since 1981:

  • Calories do count. "The new report puts a strong emphasis on getting calories under control and pays no heed to popular

diets that focus on specific nutrients, such as counting carbohydrates."

- " 'Discretionary calories,' including sweet treats," should be
reserved for "Americans who eat and exercise right and get their
nutrients without exceeding their calorie limits."

- "We need more fiber." We can get more fiber from eating complex carbohydrates, such as whole grains.

- "Most people seeking to control their weight need 60 to 90
minutes of moderate to vigorous activity daily."[7]

WHERE TO START

The book that you hold in your hands is all about first steps. This chapter has unloaded a lot of information, much of which may challenge the
way you think about your diet. How can you start applying these guidelines, which closely parallel what First Place has taught for years? In the
following chapters I lay out some practical ways you can start eating better and exercising. These chapters read more like tip sheets than an
exhaustive plan. That is intentional. Remember what you read in the
chapter on new beginnings: You must face reality and start where you are.

Notes
1. U.S. Department of Agriculture, "Revision of the Food Guidance System,"
   Backgrounder.
2. U.S. Department of Agriculture, "Revision of the Food Guidance System," *Q&As,*
   July 12, 2004.
3. Nicholas Zamiska, "New Diet Guide: Fewer Grains, More Veggies," *The Wall Street
   Journal,* August 30, 2004.
4. Ibid.
5. Stephanie Gundel, "The New Food Pyramid," *Health Beat,* September 2, 2003.
   http://depts.washington.edu/hsnews/hb/hb2003/09_02_03.html (accessed October
   22, 2004).
6. Nicholas Zamiska, "New Diet Guide: Fewer Grains, More Veggies," *The Wall Street
   Journal,* August 30, 2004.
7. Ira Dreyfuss, "New Food Pyramid Calls for More Grains, Exercise," *Lawrence Journal-
   World* (Lawrence, KS), August 28, 2004. http://www.ljworld.com/section/citynews/
   story/179743 (accessed October 22, 2004).

ABBY MELOY

Pastor's Wife
Lake City, Florida

It has been five years since I began the First Place program, and today I am one truly thankful woman. I had been at the 200-pound mark (and over) for seven years. Now my weight stays around 135 pounds and I wear size 8 clothes.

In the beginning, I did not want to try First Place. I had no desire to weigh my food or take the time to learn the measurements, but since some women at my church wanted the program—and since I was a size 18/20—I thought I'd give it a shot. After my first three-month session, I was 27 pounds lighter and I had new insights on the fact that my body is the temple of the Holy Spirit. It took me nine months and three sessions to lose 74 pounds.

My favorite Scripture used in the program is Deuteronomy 30:11: "Now what I am commanding you today is not too difficult for you or beyond your reach."

I am now truly a new creature. My new lifestyle has inspired my husband to lose 20 pounds and my 13-year-old daughter to lose 35 pounds that she needed to lose. As a result, we are able to carry out the work of our ministry with much less fatigue. I now teach others in my church the First Place program and will be forever grateful that the Lord brought it into my life.

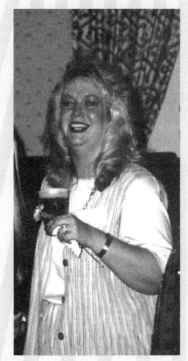

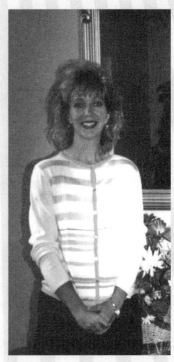

Before First Place   *Today*

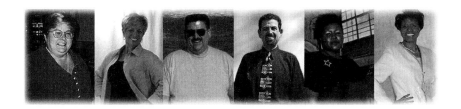

Chapter 7

A GOOD
NUTRITIONAL PLAN

*Setting a goal is not the main thing. It is deciding how you will go
about achieving it and staying with that plan.*

TOM LANDRY

Do you realize that some of the most important health decisions you
make are in the supermarket? That's right, healthy nutrition begins in
the aisles of your grocery store! How do you decide what to buy when
you shop?

- Do you purchase certain foods out of habit?
- Do you buy foods for taste or convenience?
- Do you usually choose those brands that are most familiar to
  you?
- Do you look for what's on sale or use coupons to help you
  decide?
- Do you read nutrition labels and comparison shop to help you

choose the healthiest foods?

· Are you overwhelmed by the thousands of choices in the aisles of your grocery store?

No matter how you answered these questions, you can use this helpful shopping guide and your nutrition knowledge to choose those foods that will help you reach your goals for a healthy weight and good overall health.

PLANNING TO SHOP

The best way to buy those foods that fit into your eating plan is to *plan ahead*. Planning ahead will eliminate the wasted time of having to make a second or third trip to the store. When you plan, do so for several days at a time.

· What dishes will you be preparing?
· What foods will you need for breakfast, lunch and dinner?
· Will you be eating out during the week?

Check your cupboards, refrigerator and freezer.

· Take stock of what you have, so you can use these foods first in upcoming meals.
· As you look, begin making a list of things you need from the store.

Make a list.

· Keep an ongoing list in a convenient place in your kitchen.
· Add foods, supplies and ingredients to your list as you think of them.
· Use coupons only for foods that fit into your eating plan.

- Before you go shopping, compare your grocery list with your meal plan to make sure you have listed all the items you need.

There are a few wise steps you can take before you leave for the store.

- Eat before you shop; never go to the store on an empty stomach!
- Plan on shopping during off-hours: early in the morning, late in the evening and midweek. When it's less crowded, you'll be more relaxed and have more time to make healthy decisions.
- Lace up your walking shoes so that you can pick up the pace as you shop—every bit of physical activity counts! Intentionally park a little further away from the store entrance than is necessary.

IMPLEMENTING THE PLAN

And there are certain things you can do when you step inside the store.

- Rely on your list to help you stick to your shopping plan.
- First, walk around the outside aisles of your store. That's where you'll find the fresh produce, dairy products, baked goods, fresh meats, poultry and fish. Save for last the inside aisles, which contain more processed foods.
- Do not select or purchase foods that don't fit into your eating plan, no matter how tempting the packaging appears.
- Use food labels to help you make the healthiest choices. Avoid or limit foods with the following terms in the ingredients list: beef fat, coconut oil, lard, butter, hardened shortening, palm kernel oil, chicken fat, hydrogenated shortening and palm oil.

RENA SCHAEFFER

Atlanta, Texas

My weight began to increase as my lifestyle changed after the birth of my two children. They were born 16 months apart, so I stayed busy raising babies for about three years. Much of the 1980s was spent concentrating on being a good mom. I forgot about taking care of me.

Toward the end of the 1980s, I lost my mother, my father and my step-father in a period of less than one year. The grief was coupled with increased stress levels as my family moved to a new home and we purchased a new business—on the same day! My weight continued to increase.

The fast-paced 1990s rolled in as my kids stayed busy in school and I stayed home. Before I knew it, my weight had skyrocketed to 219 pounds. I was miserable and unhappy with my physical appearance. One day I looked in the mirror and decided to make a change. That night I told a dear friend that I was going to lose weight. I began to lose a little as I exercised and tried to eat fewer sweets and more green salads. Before long I had lost 40 pounds. It was not easy, but I felt successful.

I knew I had more weight to lose but had no idea how to achieve it. I was standing in the produce isle of my favorite grocery store when a friend invited me to a First Place meeting—the meeting was that night. I went, and my life has never been the same.

I lost an additional 40 pounds in one three-month session. It can be done! With God's help, I followed the program as it was designed. I remember the struggles I experienced as I would walk on the track, headphones on, listening to a First Place audiocassette. I would cry out loud to God and ask Him to help me eat better and lose weight. The battle was His, and He proved faithful.

I began leading a First Place group in 1996, at the age of 42. I have seen many people become success stories as they change their lives, begin to exercise and learn to eat healthier foods.

Watching people change their lives and live healthier is exciting. I made a decision in 2000 to return to college. I wanted to study nutrition and learn more about how to help people achieve good health. I began attending classes at a local community college. After two semesters of general chemistry my first year, I knew that with God nothing was impossible!

I am taking Kansas State University Distance Education courses and studying dietetics and should receive my degree soon after this book is published. Following a 12-month internship I will sit for the registered dietician exam.

Mostly women attend my First Place groups. When I open a new session, I show everyone a picture of myself at 219 pounds. It never fails: They have a hard time believing I am really the one in the picture. It gets their attention. I have been where they are, and I know and understand their struggle.

One woman came to the first session after eating a large Snickers bar and drinking a 16-ounce Dr. Pepper. She knew it would be her last. That woman was successful and has kept off the weight she lost. Another woman had never had a weight problem until she reached age 50. She, too, has been successful and made changes to improve her health and lifestyle. Another woman could not walk to her mailbox at the time she came to the first meeting. Today she has lost approximately 25 pounds and walks around the block and rides a stationary bicycle.

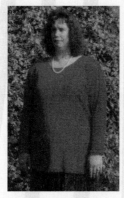

Before First Place

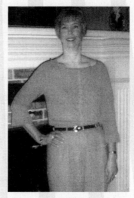

Today

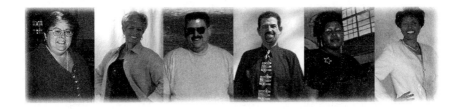

Chapter 8

HEALTHY FOOD CHOICES

The first step towards getting somewhere is to decide that you are not going to stay where you are.

JOHN PIERPONT MORGAN

As a way to help you get a jump start to a better diet, in this chapter we will look at some healthy food choices you can make throughout the day. This is a quick scan of some highlights rather than a comprehensive revamping of your overall diet. If you are busy or not sure that any change in your food intake will help or is possible, start here. Once you see and feel the difference just a few changes make, you may just want to know more and take additional steps. When you do that, you will see bigger differences in your weight and your health. Better living starts with you. It is your choice to make each day.

IN THE MORNING

Do you really need to eat breakfast? Yes. No nutritional substitute exists for a good breakfast. Having a good breakfast has two major advantages.

Breakfast generally provides important nutrients, especially vitamin C, calcium and riboflavin. Additionally, you will want your children to have breakfast. Skipping the first meal of the day may reduce a child's attention span and performance at school, especially his or her problem-solving ability. Breakfast provides fuel for the morning hours and helps rebuild glycogen stores depleted during the night's fast. A child has approximately 12-15 hours of glycogen stored in the liver and muscles, and if breakfast is skipped, then the body must convert protein to glycogen.

A healthy breakfast provides the protein a person needs to start the day no matter your age. Protein is needed in the body to perform other vital functions, and using it to make glycogen causes abnormal stress on the body. Research indicates that people who skip breakfast may be cutting their life expectancy up to five years.

Here are some suggestions for a healthy breakfast:

- Choose toast, a small (or half) bagel or English muffin with a small amount of margarine or low-fat cream cheese and jam or jelly. Add nonfat milk and fruit or fruit juice to balance out your meal.
- Cold or hot cereal with nonfat milk is a great start to any day. Top with fresh or dried fruit for added nutrition. Choose wholesome cereals with little or no added sugar and three or more grams of fiber.
- Limit eggs (two or three each week), bacon, sausage, fried potatoes, biscuits, croissants and sweet rolls. Muffins can be high in calories, fat and sugar.

A HEALTHY LUNCH

Do you take time for lunch? Our busy lifestyles often lead to lunch on the run. For many, lunch is a popular social time rather than a time to nourish the body. Some of us are so busy that we don't even take time for lunch.

The most popular lunchtime fares are sandwiches, hamburgers

and salads. The truth of the matter is that traditional sandwiches and salads may not be any lower in fat and calories than the fast-food burger!

Avoiding lunch leads to fatigue, hunger and overeating later in the day or night. Extreme hunger can also lead to cravings for junk food and binge eating. On the positive side, a nutritious lunch can give your body the fuel it needs to meet the physical and mental demands of the rest of the day. Lunchtime can also offer a much-needed break after a hard morning of work. A light, nutritious meal plus 10 to 20 minutes of moderate activity during the lunch hour is a great way to achieve good health and a healthy weight. Eating too much fat, calories and sugar may do you in for the rest of the day.

There are always a plethora of excuses for not eating a healthy lunch.

- **I don't have time!** Even if you can't stop for a relaxing lunch break, you can take a few minutes to eat some nutritious foods. It's easy to eat a sandwich, cheese and crackers, yogurt or fresh fruit—if you have prepared it ahead of time.
- **I don't need the calories!** This is *not* a good reason to skip lunch. Your body needs energy and nutrients throughout the day. Skipping meals only leads to overeating later in the day. With every meal you skip, you rob your body of important nutrients and sources for the energy needed to make it through the afternoon hours.

Examine your reasons for not eating a healthy lunch. What are some possible solutions? What are the benefits of eating a nutritious lunch? Begin making plans to make a nutritious lunch a regular part of your day.

Eating a healthy lunch is now easier than ever. Fast-food restaurants and some others now offer several nutritious and low-fat options. Of course, most menus offer selections that are high in calories, fat and cholesterol, and low in fresh fruits, vegetables and whole grains. The key is to plan ahead and order what you know is best.

BEST CHOICES FOR A HEALTHY LUNCH

- A fresh salad with low-fat dressing (on the side, please!) and an assortment of colorful vegetables, grilled chicken, grilled chicken sandwich (hold the mayo!), bean and cheese burrito (go easy on the cheese and add extra lettuce and tomato!), small hamburger or baked potato (toppings on the side!) are all good choices. All these meals have fewer than 400 calories and 30 percent or less fat.
- Deli sandwiches can be a healthy choice. Choose lean meats such as turkey, ham or roast beef. Ask for mustard or light mayonnaise. Ask for less meat (usually half the typical serving), more lettuce, tomato and other vegetables, and whole-grain bread. Hold the chips or fries.
- Pizza can be a good choice if you choose carefully. Stick to vegetable pizza and ask for less cheese and more sauce and vegetables. Limit yourself to one or two slices of thin-crust pizza. Eat a salad, too—with low-fat dressing on the side!
- Pick out three or four restaurants where you know you can get healthy foods. Suggest to friends and colleagues that you eat at these places when you eat out for lunch.

WORST BETS FOR A HEALTHY LUNCH

- A hamburger and fries, a tuna-salad sandwich or a chicken Caesar salad can supply half of the fat and calories recommended for an entire day. The typical deli-style sandwich piled with meat, mayonnaise and cheese—and bacon if it's a club sandwich—is not any better.
- Is salad a healthy choice? It depends on what you put in/on it. A ladle of regular salad dressing contains four tablespoons—

nearly 300 calories of fat or half of your recommended daily intake.
- Fried foods—French fries, fried chicken and fish, burgers, tacos and so on—should not be a regular part of the lunchtime meal. Frying can double the fat and calories.
- Portion sizes can be two to three times what you need—split a meal with a companion or take some home to eat for another meal.

—Jody Wilkinson, M.D., M.S., physician, exercise physiologist and director of the Cooper Institute Weight Management Research Center, Dallas, Texas.

PACK A LUNCH

Packing a healthy lunch starts with planning. A healthy brown-bag lunch starts in the grocery store. Plan ahead to buy a variety of nutritious foods that you enjoy and are convenient for you to prepare and pack along. When preparing your lunch, remember the key principles of variety, balance and moderation.

- You'll need an assortment of plastic containers, plastic bags and maybe even a thermos. An insulated lunch bag or cooler can keep foods cool if you don't have access to a refrigerator.
- Canned and frozen fruits, vegetables and beans can be placed in individual-sized plastic containers. You can do the same with soups. Add your own seasonings when packing. Your meal is now ready to heat in a microwave when you're ready.
- Take along low-fat dairy foods. Milk can be kept cool in a thermos and yogurt can stay at room temperature for several hours. Mix canned fruit or fresh vegetables with cottage

cheese in a plastic container.

- Keep plenty of your favorite fruits and vegetables on hand wherever you are. If they need cutting or peeling, do it the night before. Better yet, prepare them as soon as you come home from the grocery store. Store them away in plastic bags or containers so that they're ready to go when you are.
- Make a sandwich with lean meat and fresh vegetables the night before. Place it in a sandwich container or plastic bag, and it will be ready to go when you leave in the morning.
- Make lunch quick and easy by bringing leftovers. Most leftovers can be easily reheated in a microwave. When cooking at home, make extra portions and store the extras individually for a ready-to-serve lunch.
- Packing your own lunch also saves money; it's much cheaper to pack your own than to eat out. The savings over an entire year could pay for a health-club membership or home-exercise equipment!
- Always have enjoyable standbys when you find yourself short on time or choices. Dried and canned soups and fruits, crackers, peanut butter, oatmeal, cereal, bagels and energy bars can be kept on hand in a pantry or desk drawer for a quick and easy lunch anytime.

AN EASY-TO-USE RESTAURANT GUIDE

Eating out is a great way to spend time with family and friends and enjoy good food. Believe it or not, you can dine out without blowing your healthy eating plan! The key is having a plan and sticking with it.

Check Out What's on the Menu
Menus are full of food clues, if you know what to look for. Here is a list of terms often used in menus.

Less Fat	More Fat
Baked or broiled	Fried
Poached	Breaded
Grilled	Sautéed (in butter or oil)
Tomato sauce	Alfredo or cream sauce
Roasted	Casserole
Steamed	Prime

Big portions are a problem when eating out. Almost any restaurant meal can be a good choice if you don't eat all of it. The key to controlling portions is to have a plan before you order. Try the following helpful tips:

- Choose single items and side dishes rather than complete meals.
- Ask for a to-go box before you eat your meal. Choose what you need and immediately box the rest.
- Share a dish with a companion or plan to eat smaller portions of dishes that are higher in calories, fat and sugar.

SURVIVAL TIPS

- When eating out with family and friends, tell them in advance that you plan to eat healthily. Order what you know is best for you and don't allow yourself to be tempted by others.
- If you know a meal will be high in calories and fat, choose more healthy foods during the rest of the day. Don't skip any meals!
- Start your meal with a fresh salad and broth-based soup to help control your appetite. Better yet, when you know you are dining out, eat a piece of fruit or drink a glass of nonfat milk before you go.
- When eating at a buffet, plan in advance to choose healthier foods. Fill up on low-fat items such as fruits, vegetables, low-fat breads and crackers and lean meats.

- Choose baked, broiled or grilled chicken (without the skin), fish or small portions of other lean meats. Limit fried and prime cuts of meat and heavy sauces.

- Pastas with tomato-based sauces and fresh vegetables are good choices. Limit cream- or cheese-based sauces. When you order, ask that the sauce be served on the side.

- When eating out, you can burn off a few extra calories by parking your car a few blocks away and walking. Make a plan to go for a walk before or after eating.

YOUR SALT INTAKE

When it comes to health, sodium (salt) has drawn a considerable amount of attention because of its relationship to high blood pressure.

WHAT ABOUT DESSERT?

- First, ask yourself whether you're really hungry. If you're not, then save dessert for another time. If you are hungry, the best choices include fresh fruit, sorbet, frozen yogurt, sherbet or angel food cake with a fruit topping.

- Desserts aren't always off-limits; just keep your overall goal in mind. If you know in advance that you want dessert, plan to split your favorite treat with a companion. Another option is to slowly eat your dessert and to eat only a few bites.

—Dr. Jody Wilkinson

High blood pressure is a leading risk factor for heart attack, stroke and kidney disease. Scientists have discovered that some people's blood pressure is very sensitive to excess sodium in the diet.

Because high blood pressure is such a serious health problem, the current U.S. Dietary Guidelines call for Americans to choose a diet moderate in salt and sodium. Most of the salt in the American diet comes from processed foods however, not the saltshaker. Only about 15 percent of the sodium in the average diet is added in the kitchen or at the table. The top sources of salt in the diet include processed meats, prepackaged meals, fast foods, canned and dried soups, cheese, salted snack foods and certain condiments. The best way to learn how much sodium is in a food is to read the label. For a food to be labeled "low sodium," it must contain less than 140 milligrams of sodium. A good rule of thumb is to choose foods that provide less than 5 percent of the daily value for sodium. Foods that provide over 300 milligrams per serving are particularly high in sodium. For a single food item to carry the term "healthy" on the label, it must contain 360 or fewer milligrams of sodium per serving. Here are some foods particularly high in sodium:

- Canned and dried soups—1 cup contains 600-1,300 milligrams.
- Prepackaged meals (i.e., frozen dinners)—8 ounces contain 500-1,570 milligrams.
- Soy sauce—1 tablespoon contains 1,030 milligrams.
- Salted popcorn—2½ cups contain 330 milligrams.
- Processed cheese and cheese spreads—1 ounce contains 340-450 milligrams.
- Cured ham—3 ounces contain 1,025 milligrams.

While we're born with a preference for sweet tastes, salt is an acquired taste. Many people find that after cutting down on salt, many foods that they used to enjoy taste too salty. Cut down gradually to give your taste buds time to adapt. To be sure you consume no more than 2,400 milligrams of sodium per day, try these helpful tips:

- Choose foods that are naturally low in sodium, such as fresh fruits and vegetables.
- Break the habit of adding salt during cooking—there's no reason to salt cooking water—or at the table.
- Rinse canned meats, legumes and vegetables under cold water to remove excess salt.
- Eat a variety of foods during a single meal to stimulate the taste buds.
- Eat meals slowly and savor the flavor and aroma of each bite.
- Cut the salt called for in most recipes by half (or more).

- For meals with dried seasoning packets, use half or less of the packet to cut down on the sodium.
- Learn to season foods with herbs, spices, fruit juice and flavored vinegars.
- Limit processed meats, such as ham, bacon, hot dogs and lunch meats.
- Limit high-salt condiments, such as soy sauce, steak sauce, barbecue sauce, mustard and ketchup.
- Buy reduced-salt or low-salt snack foods.
- Limit consumption of olives, pickles, relishes and many salad dressings, which are loaded with salt.
- When eating out, ask for meals to be prepared with less salt, ask for sauces to be served on the side and avoid using the saltshaker.

WHY DO I CRAVE SALT?

Most likely you want more salt because your body has become accustomed to a high level of sodium intake. Don't imagine that your craving reflects a true need. People who use little salt have less sodium in their bodies and don't crave it. In fact, they prefer less-salty food. When a person who is used to a lot of salt reduces his or her salt intake, the body at first craves it, but as the sodium level declines, so does the craving for salt. This craving normally subsides in about two weeks.

—*Dr. Richard Couey*

HERBS AND SPICES

Adding herbs, spices or other flavorings is a great way to make tasty dishes that are low in sodium. You'll have to experiment to find out what works best for you. Here are some tips on using and storing herbs and spices:

- Read the label; some premixed spices contain salt.

- Store herbs and spices in a cool, dark place and in tight containers. Avoid heat, moisture and light.
- Date dry herbs and spices when you buy them; their shelf life is about one year.
- Test the freshness of herbs by rubbing them between your fingers and checking the aroma.
- Crumble dry herbs between your fingers before using to release more flavor.
- Liquid brings out the flavor of dried herbs and spices.
- If you use fresh herbs, store them in a plastic bag in the refrigerator. Before using, wash and pat dry.
- For soups and stews—dishes that have to cook awhile—add herbs and spices toward the end of cooking.
- For chilled dishes or meats, the earlier you add the herbs and spices, the better the flavor.
- When trying new herbs and spices, add them gradually to the dish—you can always add more.

SEASONING IDEAS FOR MEAT AND VEGETABLES

Beef	Bay leaf, dry mustard, marjoram, nutmeg, onion, pepper, sage, thyme
Fish	Curry powder, dill, dry mustard, lemon juice, marjoram, paprika, pepper
Poultry	Ginger, marjoram, oregano, paprika, rosemary, sage, tarragon, sage, thyme
Carrots	Cinnamon, cloves, marjoram, nutmeg, rosemary, sage
Corn	Cumin, curry powder, green pepper, onion, paprika, parsley
Green beans	Dill, curry powder, lemon juice, marjoram, oregano, tarragon, thyme
Peas	Basil, dill, ginger, marjoram, onion, parsley, sage

Potatoes	Basil, dill, garlic, onion, paprika, parsley, rosemary, sage
Squash	Allspice, basil, cinnamon, curry powder, ginger, marjoram, nutmeg, onion, rosemary, sage
Tomatoes	Basil, bay leaf, dill, marjoram, onion, oregano, parsley, pepper, thyme

WHY DO I CRAVE CAFFEINE?

Most adults and senior adults (approximately 80 percent) consume caffeine in some form. Caffeine is the most popular drug in America. It occurs naturally in more than 60 plants and trees that have been cultivated by humans since the beginning of recorded history. Whether people get their caffeine in coffee or tea, cocoa, headache remedies or soft drinks, nearly everyone ingests at least some caffeine daily. Most adult Americans begin their day with coffee or tea; others, including many children, get their morning started with a cola (12 percent of all soft drinks are now consumed at breakfast). The average American coffee drinker consumes three cups a day. Yet many people worry about caffeine's side effects. Caffeine is a mind-altering drug, and if consumed in sufficient amounts, it can bring on the jitters. Caffeine also has been accused of causing pancreatic cancer, heart disease, breast disease, high blood pressure, high blood cholesterol levels and birth defects. But does it? Let's review what the latest research tells us.

Kicking the Habit
If you are a healthy adult who enjoys coffee or tea, no evidence suggests that caffeine will do you any harm, if consumed in moderation. Most people should limit their intake to no more than two caffeinated beverages per day. If it gives you a lift or a reason to relax in the mid-afternoon, you should not deprive yourself of caffeine's benefits. If you think caffeine may be robbing you of a sound night's sleep, try cutting out caffeine in the evening. If you get jittery and nervous from it at any time of day, cut back consumption.

Caffeine is a habit-forming drug, and some heavy coffee and tea drinkers may experience withdrawal symptoms, such as drowsiness, headache, lethargy, irritability and nausea, 12 to 16 hours after their final doses. Even passing up the regular after-dinner cup can cause a morning-after headache. Such symptoms can be avoided simply by cutting back gradually. You can switch to decaffeinated coffee or other caffeine-free beverages, which, however, also may have unwanted side effects.

Despite the lack of clear evidence linking caffeine to most of the evils that have been attributed to caffeine, many doctors suggest caution. Doctors often advise pregnant or nursing women, children and people with heart disease to abstain from caffeine or to at least restrict their intake to 200 milligrams daily. People with heart disease who are subject to arrhythmias should avoid caffeine altogether. Anyone who has suffered a heart attack should avoid caffeine for the first several weeks afterward, because of its arhythmogenic effects. Anyone who is prone to coffee nerves would be advised to cut down or eliminate coffee from his or her diet.

Caffeine and Blood Pressure

The rapidly beating heart some people feel after drinking coffee or tea has nothing to do with a persistent rise in blood pressure. After reviewing the results of 17 studies, scientists concluded that coffee, tea and other caffeinated beverages do not cause any a lasting increase in blood pressure. To be sure, the blood pressure of people who do not consume caffeine on a regular basis may rise slightly and temporarily on a particular day when they do happen to take in some coffee, tea or soft drink. But this effect is usually short-lived, lasting only about a day at most.

A word of caution: Individuals with irregular heartbeats may experience disturbances in heart rhythm when they drink caffeinated beverages. In severe cases, these disturbances can be life threatening.

—Dr. Richard Couey

MARK GUTIERREZ

Chino, California

When I was a little boy, I was chubby. It didn't really bother me until I got into junior high school. That's when I started my first diet—I was only 13. By the age of 37, I'd been on countless diets—and they all worked. I would lose weight, but sooner or later, I would gain it back, and even more. In my mind I conceded that I would be fat forever.

In 1998, my church started a program called First Place. I remember thinking to myself, *Oh! That won't work.* But I was so desperate, discouraged and angry that I was willing to give it a try. I thought that if I at least lost some weight, things would get better.

On January 11, 1999, I started First Place and it quickly became a life-changing journey. I felt overwhelmed that first night, but I also was encouraged to start where I was. I must have done something right, because in the first week I lost 13 pounds. After a couple of weeks I started exercising, which is something I'd never before done—on any diet. Two or three more weeks passed and I began to read a devotional Bible and work on the Bible study. After six weeks I reached my session goal of losing 35 pounds (First Place encourages participants to set a weight-loss goal) and was told to keep going (and keep losing). By the end of the first 13 weeks I had lost 57 pounds. By Christmas of that year I was 120 pounds lighter.

I wish I could say that I've kept the 120 pounds off, but the truth is that the lifestyle-change part of the program has taken years to sink in. I gained back more than 50 of the pounds that I had lost. I almost lost hope and I wanted to drop out, but I recommitted to the program and I again began to lose weight. A few months later I picked up *Back on Track,* by Carole Lewis. That book motivated me to get moving again. At this writing, it's been about nine months since I first read that book and I'm down almost 30 pounds. I'm less than 10 pounds from that 120 I had originally lost—and I'm committed to reaching my weight-loss goal.

There are good days and bad days. Sometimes I will eat right and at other times I will not, but when I slip up I get right back on track. I've also made fitness my life desire and try to keep learning about it. However, I don't put much effort in keeping up with the latest fads; rather, I stick with the basics. The basics are things that we don't really have to be taught, such as eating a balanced diet that includes a variety of foods, and common-sense actions like exercising regularly. These are the things I must do consistently if this weight loss is going to last me a lifetime.

Over the years God has changed my attitude about food. Before coming to First Place, I never drank water, nor did I eat vegetables or fruit. It was a diet of meat and carbs for this guy. Now I drink far more than those eight glasses of water that are recommended for each of us to have each day, and I enjoy eating all kinds of vegetables and fruits. God has made eating these healthy foods enjoyable for me, and I have learned to be content with smaller portions. I'm not saying that I don't enjoy an occasional greasy cheeseburger and order of onion rings, but that is no longer my regular meal.

I was challenged to look in the Bible and find a life-defining verse. I prayed and came upon 1 Corinthians 9:24: "Do you not know that in a race all the runners run, but only one gets the prize? Run in such a way as to get the prize." A couple weeks after I found that verse God gave me a second Scripture: "Brothers, I do not consider myself yet to have taken hold of it. But one thing I do: Forgetting what is behind and straining toward what is ahead" (Phil. 3:13).

I refuse to give up in the midst of this race I'm running. I know that God has some great plans for my life, so I must persevere. I desire to serve God as long as I can. I thank God for First Place and my new healthy lifestyle. First Place changed my life—it took my broken spirit and restored hope, and it helped give me a brighter future.

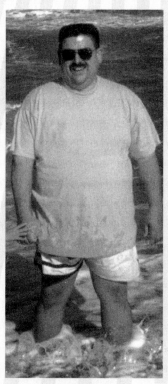

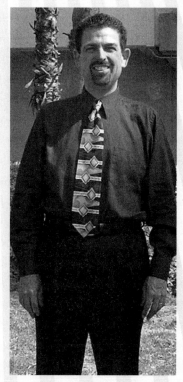

Before First Place   *Today*

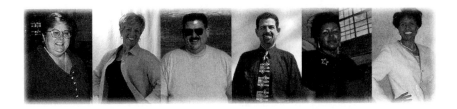

C h a p t e r   9

PORTION CONTROL

We are able to conquer our weaknesses and maintain self-control when we focus on putting our hope and faith in Christ Jesus rather than our own abilities.

PASTOR JACK GRAHAM

Serving sizes may be one of the biggest factors causing the rising rate of obesity in this country. When it comes to food these days, bigger is better. Undoubtedly you hear the terms "super meal deals," "supersize" and "50 percent more" when you're out eating or shopping. In many restaurants one meal is sometimes big enough to feed a family. Even too much of the right foods can make you gain weight. Learning appropriate portion sizes for different foods may be one of the most important skills you can learn when it comes to achieving and maintaining your healthy weight. It's a skill that takes time and practice to develop.

MASTERING PORTION CONTROL

- Use the right tools. Make sure you use measuring cups and spoons and a food scale to help you learn about the portion sizes you eat. These tools allow you to compare what you *really* eat with what you *should* eat. Measure all the foods you eat to learn about common servings.

- Try eating with smaller plates and bowls. This will help you avoid serving portions that are too large. It also makes smaller portions look bigger.
- Cut foods, especially meat, into smaller pieces. This also gives the appearance of more food and can help the meal last longer.
- Buy meats and cheese that are already cut in appropriate serving sizes.
- Get out of the habit of eating everything on your plate, especially at restaurants. Learn to stop eating before you're full; it's okay to leave some food behind. It's also okay to split a meal with a companion.

CONTROLLING MEAT, POULTRY AND FISH PORTIONS

One of the areas in which calories can easily add up unnoticed is the meat group. The recommended serving size for meat is 3 ounces. Unfortunately, we've gotten used to eating two to three times this amount. This is especially challenging when eating in restaurants. The average portion of meat served when dining out is 6 to 10 ounces. Remember, too, that restaurants don't always offer the leanest cuts of meat. With all of this in mind, it is a good idea to learn how to estimate a 3-ounce portion of meat.

3 OUNCES OF MEAT, POULTRY OR FISH= ¼ OF THE PLATE

CARBOHYDRATES= ¾ OF THE PLATE

- Dinner-plate rule—Imagine a standard dinner plate divided in quarters. Your meat serving should only fill one-quarter of your plate. This means the other three-quarters should consist of complex carbohydrates (one-fourth starch and one-half vegetables or fruit).

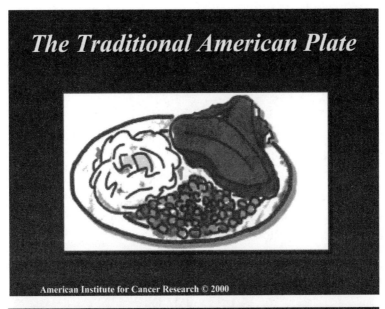

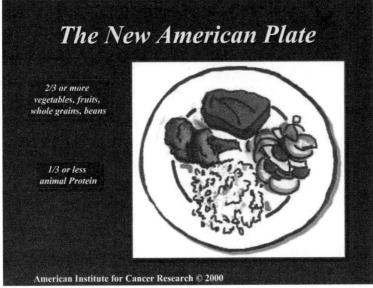

• Deck-of-cards rule—This is an old favorite when trying to estimate 3-ounce portions of meat. A 3-ounce portion of meat should be no thicker and no wider than a standard deck of cards (or about the size of an audiocassette).

- Lady's-palm rule—Three ounces of meat should fit nicely in the palm of an average-sized lady's palm.
- Checkbook rule—Three ounces of grilled fish is the size of a checkbook.
- Eyeball rule—This is a simple rule of thumb that is easy to apply: If it looks too big, it probably is!

When grocery shopping, keep in mind that chicken breasts are typically closer to 5 or 6 ounces each. Individual filet mignons, although they look small, are at least 6- to 8-ounce portions. It's a good idea to plan on cutting these portions in half before preparing. Eating a couple of ounces more than you should can add at least 100 calories!

SHORTCUTS FOR ESTIMATING PORTION SIZES

The key to moderation is controlling portion size. To achieve and maintain a healthy weight, learn to put into practice the concept of "serving size." Use measuring cups, spoons and scales until you know appropriate portion sizes by heart. Following are some practical examples from the American Dietetics Association to help you estimate portion sizes when those tools aren't available:

- A medium potato is the size of a computer mouse.
- An average bagel is the size of a hockey puck.
- A cup of fruit is the size of a baseball.
- A cup of lettuce is four leaves.
- One ounce of cheese is the size of four dice.
- One ounce of snack foods, such as pretzels, is one handful.

MARTHA ROGERS

Houston, Texas

I wanted to lose weight—doesn't everyone? But I did not want to join a First Place group. I had commitments, I was busy, and I did not want to be hemmed in by a diet regimen. Those were my excuses. Finally, I agreed to check it out. In the first few weeks I was surprised to discover something entirely different from what I had expected. From the beginning, they made it clear that losing weight or seeing any other change in my life was up to me and would be determined by the various lifestyle choices I made. With God's help, in nine months I lost 44 pounds and reached my goal weight.

Since that time I have maintained a weight of no more than 10 pounds over that goal weight. When I do gain a few pounds, I stay on the First Place program and seek God's help.

The greatest blessing of First Place has been the Bible studies. Not only have I memorized the recommended verses each week, but I have memorized additional verses as well. At certain times, these verses have given me exactly what I needed to face a particular problem or test. Those verses have taken me through two cancer surgeries and my husband's heart attacks and surgery, and now they are helping us cope with our grandson's life-threatening illness.

The first year after I reached my goal, Carole Lewis asked me to be a First Place leader. I jumped at the chance and have been heading up groups almost steadily since then. Leading a group helps me stay focused and gives me the opportunity to encourage so many others.

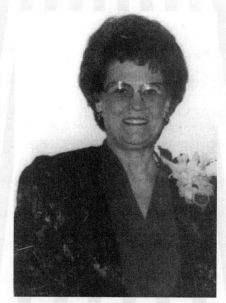

Before First Place

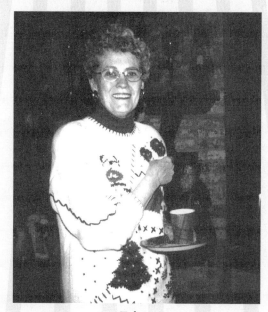

Today

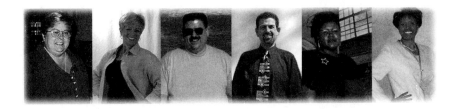

Chapter 10

ON THE RUN

Do you not know that in a race all the runners run, but only one
gets the prize? Run in such a way as to get the prize.

1 CORINTHIANS 9:24

It is true: As you grow older, time moves faster, or at least it seems that way. One of the most common reasons given by people who need to lose weight and improve their health but do not is that they do not have the time. Kids, work, traffic jams, bills to pay, soccer games, in-laws, housework, homework—you name it, and it will demand more and more of our time each day. So how do we make headway in the midst of our busy lives? In this chapter I have compiled some jump-start suggestions that will get you moving in the right direction.

FAST-FOOD FARE

Eating in the fast-food lane has become a way of life for many of us. Life has us on the go, so we have to eat on the go. Why do people choose to eat fast foods? *Taste, convenience* and *price* top the list. These reasons are important, but *good nutrition* and *health* should be at the top of your list.

What foods do you think of when you think fast food? Burgers and fries, fried chicken, tacos and burritos, and soft drinks? A fast-food meal can easily top 1,000 calories and give you a day's worth of fat, cholesterol and sodium. Believe it or not, you can also make healthy fast-food choices. Today, most fast-food restaurants offer a variety of foods, such as grilled chicken, salads, baked potatoes and deli-style sandwiches. Of course, fresh fruits and vegetables are hard to find. The key is to plan ahead and be prepared to make healthy choices. Look for ways to trim fat, cut calories and add variety whenever you can. Always keep your goals of a healthy weight and good nutrition in mind. Here are some helpful tips—pick the ones that will work best for you.

PRACTICAL TIPS FOR EATING ON THE RUN

- Order individual items rather than the special meal deal. One item that is higher in calories and fat may be okay, but add fries and a soft drink and you may double the calories and fat.
- Watch out for words such as "deluxe," "supersize" or "jumbo." Order the regular or small size instead. A single slice of cheese on a small burger adds calcium. Think nutrition—add the cheese and cut the fries.
- Choose sandwiches with grilled chicken or fish, or lean roast beef, turkey or ham. Ask for low-fat toppings such as mustard or low-fat salad dressing instead of mayonnaise or special sauce.
- If you're having fast food for one meal, choose healthier foods the rest of the day. Don't forget your fruits and vegetables. You can even carry a piece of fruit with you to eat with your meal.

Lettuce Works
- Beware—salads can have more calories, fat and sodium than a burger and fries! Limit items such as cheese, croutons, bacon,

eggs, nuts and creamy salad dressings. Add more vegetables instead.

- Choose the right greens. Many people think they are eating well when they choose iceberg lettuce (often found on fast-food hamburgers and in dinner salads at restaurants). The truth is that although iceberg lettuce is full of water and can be a source of vitamin K, beyond that it has very little nutritional value. Romaine and other leafy greens are better, especially if you consume large amounts. Fresh spinach is the best nutritional choice.
- Always order salad dressing on the side. Use the low-fat dressing whenever possible. Salsa and low-fat cottage cheese are also good choices. Add flavor with fresh fruits, peppers and other vegetables.
- Limit special salads such as potato, macaroni, tuna and chicken. These salads are often made with mayonnaise or high-fat salad dressing. Choose coleslaw or bean salad made with vinaigrette instead.

Potato Toppings

- Plain baked potatoes are low in calories and fat and are a good source of fiber and vitamin C. Limit toppings such as butter, cheese, bacon and sour cream.
- Healthier choices include small amounts of margarine and low-fat sour cream. Other good toppings include low-fat cottage cheese, plain yogurt and salsa. Pack on the nutrition by adding lots of fresh vegetables.

Fast-Food Olé

- Choose grilled chicken (without the skin), beans or vegetables instead of beef or cheese on tostadas, tacos or burritos. Ask for your bean burrito to be prepared with less cheese. Order soft tortillas rather than fried.
- Go easy on—or abstain from—cheese, sour cream and guacamole. Add more lettuce, tomatoes and salsa.

The Orient Express

- Asian take-out is one fast-food option that offers a variety of vegetables. Watch out, however, since portion sizes can be large! Make a plan to split a dish with a companion or save some for another meal.
- Ask before you order. Many Asian dishes include fried meats. Order steamed rice instead of fried rice; forego the fried egg roll and ask for extra vegetables.

The Pizza Plan

- Choose thin crust over thick crust or deep dish.
- Avoid meats such as ground beef and pepperoni. These meats are higher in fat and sodium. Instead, ask for extra tomato sauce, fresh vegetables and less cheese.
- Limit yourself to one or two slices.
- Order a salad. A healthy salad will add variety and nutrition to your meal.

Drink Up

- Choose low-fat milk or natural fruit juice to drink. This will boost the nutrition of any fast-food meal. Water is always a good choice!
- Remember that some milk shakes can equal the calories and fat of an entire meal. Keep this in mind, and cut back in other areas if you order a shake.

A Healthy Beginning

- If breakfast is most often your fast-food meal, choose a plain bagel, toast or English muffin with jelly, jam or low-fat cream cheese. Skip the croissant and biscuits, which are high in fat and calories.
- Cold or hot cereals with nonfat milk, pancakes without butter or plain scrambled eggs are also good choices. Limit high-fat meats such as bacon and sausage and watch out for fried potatoes.

BASIC GUIDELINES FOR HEALTHY EATING

Some of this information is noted in more detail in chapter 8; here's a list to review that will help you make healthy food choices when you're eating on the run.

- Never skip meals. Your body needs food throughout the day for energy. Start your day with a nutritious breakfast and don't skip lunch. Every meal you miss robs your body of important nutrients. Also, skipping meals will make it more likely that you'll overeat later.
- Prepare and take your own food. You're much more likely to eat healthy meals and snacks if you prepare them yourself. The key is planning ahead.

  - ✓ Healthy eating at work begins at the grocery store. Make a list of foods you enjoy and that are easy for you to bring to work. Choose fresh, canned or dried fruits, raw or canned vegetables, lean sandwich meats, low-fat crackers, bean or broth-based soups, low-fat milk and yogurt.
  - ✓ Cook extra portions with evening meals and pack the leftovers for work—homemade fast food.
  - ✓ If you don't have a refrigerator at work, bring an ice cooler or insulated lunch bag. Buy plastic containers in which you can store foods and beverages.
  - ✓ Store healthy snacks in your desk drawer, briefcase or car. Low-fat versions of crackers, graham crackers, cookies and bagels; fresh or dried fruit; cereal; popcorn and instant oatmeal are great choices.

- When you eat out, choose your restaurants and your meals carefully.

✓Watch your portion sizes; they are usually much more than you need.

✓Split your meal with a companion or box some of it up and bring it home.

✓Avoid fried foods and dishes cooked with heavy sauces or a lot of cheese. Choose bean or broth-based soups, baked or grilled chicken, fresh salads with low-fat dressing, steamed vegetables, sandwiches with lean meat and fresh fruit.

✓Find two or three restaurants where you know you can make healthy choices; recommend these when eating out.

BE MORE PHYSICALLY ACTIVE

Fit physical activity into your workday whenever you can. Even 5 to 10 minutes of activity done throughout the day can improve your health and fitness.

- Schedule activity into your day just like you do important meetings.
- Park your car farther away from your office building.
- Take the stairs instead of the elevator.
- Use the bathroom on at least the next floor up or across the building.
- Hand-deliver messages rather than use office mail, the computer or telephone.
- Take 10- to 15-minute walking breaks.
- Stand up and do some stretching while you're talking on the phone.
- Buy some handheld weights or elastic exercise bands to use in your office.
- Go for a walk during your lunch hour.
- Start a walking group or aerobic dance class at work.

- Make time for physical activity when you travel—walk in the airport between flights.
- Talk to your company about purchasing a few pieces of exercise equipment.

REDUCE STRESS

You may not be able to eliminate the stress of your job, but you can learn to handle it in more positive ways. Here are some tips to help you reduce and respond more positively to the stress that you may experience on the job. Stress often begins before you arrive at work—running late, taking care of personal responsibilities and fighting traffic.

- Get organized; do most of your preparation the night before.
- Be sure to get enough sleep. Most people need seven to nine hours of sleep every night. Discover how much sleep you need and try to get it every night.
- Arrange your schedule so that you can avoid driving in heavy traffic.
- Leave your home early enough so that you're not rushed.
- Take time to relax before you leave for work or while you're in the car: Breathe deeply, relax your muscles, pray or listen to relaxing music or the Bible on cassette.
- At work, once or twice a day take 10 or 15 minutes to relax and organize the rest of your day.
- Prioritize your daily and weekly activities.
- Learn to recognize things that are less important or not important at all.
- Schedule time for yourself.
- Focus on one thing at a time.
- Learn to say "No!" or "I need help!"
- Personalize your workspace with pictures and special messages.
- Avoid cigarette smoke and limit caffeine intake.

- Friends, coworkers and family can offer encouragement and support during stressful times. Look for ways to share responsibilities with others. Think of specific things people can do to help you reduce your stress.
- Set aside time each week to discuss issues, plans, schedules and responsibilities with your family, friends and coworkers. Make this a time for teamwork and positive problem solving.
- Make sure you're making time to enjoy yourself outside of work. You need to get away and take time for yourself and loved ones.

NANCY WINNIFORD

Anchorage, Alaska

I began to be weight-conscious when I was 14. My mom was very over-weight, and she often tried different diets. Sometimes I did them with her, convinced that I, too, was overweight. Significant to this part of the story is that many years later, when I was an adult, God told me to get out my old photo albums. While I looked at a photo of myself at 16, He asked me to objectively evaluate if the girl in the picture (me) was over-weight. In all honesty I had to say no. I was greatly surprised at what lies the devil can get us to believe about ourselves!

When I was in my twenties, I discovered that God could help me to choose what to eat and what not to eat. I learned a lot from Him, but I came short of letting Him be totally in charge. I learned to love exercise, to watch my diet and to keep my weight within a certain range. That all worked fine while I was single.

At 40, I got married and I began to gain weight. So did my husband. I told myself a lie. I convinced myself that it was OK to gain a little weight after 40. Before we adopted our first child, I gained 10 pounds. Then we adopted three more, and it became really hard to pay attention to all of our children's needs and my needs as well. I began letting my physical health slide. I exercised less. I ate more packaged foods. I ate more junk food and allowed myself to indulge in more sweets. When my husband had to work out of town for three straight summers, I gained weight as I struggled to do everything on the home front by myself. Eventually I weighed 36.5 pounds more than I had weighed when I got married.

If that was not enough, my time alone with the Lord became more and more scarce. Throughout those years I prayed, crying out to God that I needed His help. He let me get to the point where I was more than desperate before He nudged me over to a First Place booth display.

I bought the starter book and took a long time to read it. Life was still whizzing by so fast that I still felt overwhelmed. The eating part of the plan sounded hard enough, but the time commitment sounded impossible.

I prayed even harder, and slowly the Lord convinced me that I could make the time. Even though I could not find a First Place group near me, I began the program on my own at the end of January 2004. I knew I was receiving the Lord's help as I tried to incorporate all the commitments of the plan into my daily life. During the first week, I lost seven pounds. From that point on, I lost up to two pounds each week. However, what I gained was even more significant. I had always felt that everyone else's needs came first and that I could meet my own needs when everyone else was cared for. This plan gave me permission to care for me. I joined a fitness club on a three-day-per-week program. Those three days of each week, I work out on their machines. On the other days, I bike, swim, use my own stair stepper or walk for exercise. I now only take one day off from exercise.

I have profited most from the Scripture memory. Soaking in God's Word is a great way to renew my mind. I begin to think God's way. The Bible studies have helped me look at aspects of my life and eating from a different perspective. They have really been helpful.

I have been accountable to two friends who have been great. They are eagerly waiting the day I start a First Place group and they can join, too. I now call people to encourage them. I also use a prayer journal. I love to read God's Word, so it has not been hard to continue my practice of daily Bible reading.

Drinking eight glasses of water a day was already one of my disciplines. I have been pretty good about keeping a commitment record, missing only a few days here and there. I really didn't think I'd like eating the way the plan instructs, but I discovered new ways to make it workable for me.

I have now lost 32.5 pounds—4 pounds away from my goal! I'm very happy! Thank you, Jesus! I'm in a new chapter of abundant life, and I love it.

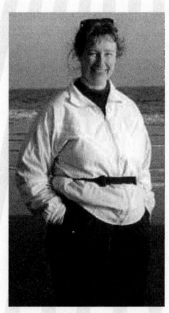

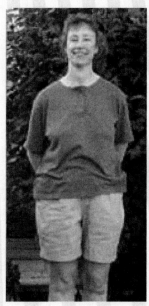

Before First Place   *Today*

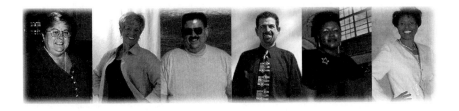

—————————— *C h a p t e r 1 1* ——————————

WATER

Worship the LORD your God, and his blessing will be on your food and water.

EXODUS 23:25

While water is not included in the Food Guide Pyramid, don't ignore it. Next to air, water is the second most important element that humans need for survival. When we keep well hydrated, we perform at our best. And we feel great, too!

Most people have heard the healthy adage: Drink eight 8-ounce glasses of water each day. Why so much? For starters, water makes up about 80 percent of our muscle mass, 60 percent of our red blood cells and more than 90 percent of our blood plasma. If we were stranded on a deserted island, we could go for weeks without food but only a few days without water.

Water does so much for the physical body. Here are just a few of its benefits:

- aids in the digestion and absorption of food and nutrients,
- helps regulate the chemical reactions in every cell of our bodies,
- transports nutrients and oxygen,
- flushes out the waste produced in normal bodily functions,

- helps to maintain a normal body temperature,
- facilitates proper bowel function and
- helps to maintain a proper fluid balance.

In the quest for healthy living, drinking plenty of water should be a top priority. In fact, if you are not currently drinking enough water, starting to do so will be one of the most significant lifestyle changes you can make.

GOOD LIQUIDS CHOICES

All fluids and some foods count toward your daily total of water. So why choose water? Water is good for us, contains no calories, is low in sodium and contains no additives or stimulants. Substituting water for calorie-containing beverages is an important step in helping to achieve and maintain a healthy body weight. Nonfat milk and 100 percent fruit juices are also good choices—they're packed with vitamins and minerals—however, we must count their calories. The caffeine in tea, soft drinks and coffee acts as a stimulant and a diuretic (i.e., causes a body to lose water); thus, caffeinated drinks are not always a good choice.

> Choose God's abundant water as your beverage of choice!

Our bodies lose about 8 to 12 ounces of water each day. To stay healthy and feel our best, we need to replace what our bodies lose. There is no magic in the number eight. Some people need a to drink a few more glasses; some fewer. Drinking water throughout the day helps keep us ahead of what we will lose.

Physical Benefits

Once you start drinking more water, your natural thirst for it will increase. With each glass you swallow, think about the physical benefits.

To make drinking water a habit, start by filling an 8-ounce measuring cup with water. In our supersized world, 8 ounces is probably not as much as you think. What size glass will you use for those 8 ounces? Another tactic is to fill a 2-quart (64-ounce) container with water each morning and by noon make sure you have only one quart left. You will be halfway to your goal!

You can keep a 2-quart pitcher of water on your desk or in your refrigerator for easy access. Additionally, you can place a water bottle in your car, take it to meetings and carry it with you when you exercise.

The Tap and the Bottle

Americans drink about 6.4 billion gallons of bottled water each year, and the amount increases each year.[1] That is about 22.6 gallons per person.[2] If drinking water from a bottle will motivate you to drink more, then bottled water is a good choice. However, don't assume that it's purer than tap water. In fact, according to the Natural Resources Defense Council (NRDC), some bottled water may not be any better than tap water—it may even *be* tap water! In a recent study, the group found that one-third of 103 tested brands of bottled water contained bacteria or other chemicals that exceed the industry's own guidelines or state purity standards.

While bottled water is safe to consume, the NRDC noted that because bottling companies tout the health benefits of their water, consumers should get greater value for their money. Since the study was released, legislation has been proposed for stricter standards on bottled water. Tap water is regulated on a national level under provisions of the Safe Drinking Water Act of 1974.

DEHYDRATION PREVENTION

During the summer, you require more water because your body loses fluids through perspiration. If you live in a dry climate, your perspiration may evaporate more quickly, so you might not sense the need to drink water, even though your body is still losing it. Don't wait for perspiration to be your warning sign to consume more liquids. The dry air in winter also increases your body's need for water. Don't wait until you feel thirsty to start drinking; stay ahead of your thirst.

In addition to thirst, early signs of dehydration include the following:

- Fatigue
- Loss of appetite
- Flushed skin
- Light-headedness and dizziness
- Muscle cramping
- Infrequent urination and urine that's dark yellow

ACTIVE LIFESTYLES

When playing sports or otherwise exerting yourself physically, pay close attention to your water intake. Make sure you drink at least 8 ounces before each activity and then another 8 ounces every 15 to 20 minutes during the

Do senior adults need to drink eight glasses of water daily?

Yes. The thirst mechanism in the body is affected as you age. Older people do not experience thirst as readily as younger people do. Their kidneys do not conserve water as well as they should during periods of dehydration. Moreover, during periods of dehydration, urine in older adults is more diluted than it is in younger adults. This dual phenomenon—the lack of thirst and the failure to conserve water in response to the body's obvious physiologic need for fluid—could lead to serious dehydration, particularly if you have a prolonged fever or diarrhea. The lack of fluid in a senior may compound the development of kidney stones and the all-too-common problem of constipation. It's a good idea to get into the habit of drinking water with each meal or in between meals, even if you don't feel the urge.

> Consumers are choosing bottled water as a refreshing, hydrating beverage and as an alternative to other drinks that may contain calories, caffeine, sugar, artificial colors, alcohol or other ingredients.
>
> —*Stephen R. Kay,*
> *International Bottled Water*
> *Association, Vice President of*
> *Communications.*

activity. You may need more if it's hot outside. To find out how much water you need to replenish your exercise losses, weigh yourself before and after exercise—the difference is mainly water. Replace one pound of weight loss with 16 ounces of water.

While the number on the scale may look better, dehydration is not a healthy way to lose weight. Avoid using a sweat suit or rubberized clothing to increase sweating during exercise. This is a dangerous practice and the weight you lose is only water—not fat! Only 25 percent of your body fat is made up of water, whereas almost 80 percent of your muscle is water. Dehydration robs your body of the water it needs.

Unless you are an endurance athlete who trains for more than an hour, drink water rather than sports drinks.

Notes

1. "Bottled Water: More Than Just a Story About Sales Growth," *International Bottled Water Association* (April 8, 2004). http://www.bottledwater.org/public/informat_main.htm (accessed October 28, 2004).
2. Ibid.

SHARON EDGEWORTH KING

Florence, South Carolina

I remember it like it was yesterday. I had read a poster that promoted First Place. Having never heard of the program, I tried to envision how weight loss and Christianity could work together. I pictured a cartoon in which the character said, "After dieting all my life, I've never lost weight or hope." That was ironic: While the first part was true for me, the second part was not. I had lost my hope.

A month earlier I had accepted defeat and resigned myself to being overweight for the rest of my life. Yet I couldn't get the impression left by the poster out of my mind. Without knowing any specifics about First Place, I decided to give it a try.

I thought, *Maybe the Christian aspect would make a difference that 22 years of dieting has not made—and just maybe I would learn something that would spare my two daughters the agony, hopelessness and defeat I had experienced while living with the problem of being overweight.*

As I write these words, it is 10 years later. I now can truly say that God granted the desire of my heart. The Christian aspect of First Place was what I had been missing, and I did learn what I needed to teach my daughters. Moreover, my hope was restored.

The program required me to examine each area of health—spiritual, physical, emotional and mental—and determine how choices I made supported the lifestyle. Not only did First Place require me to examine those choices, but First Place also taught me the changes I needed to make to bring these areas into a healthy balance.

I chose to change. In January 1995, three verses in the first Bible study (First Place promotes Bible study along with weight loss) inspired me to change. The verses helped me see the source of the problem (see Jas. 1:14) and that the temptation of food could be overcome if I looked to God (see 1 Cor. 10:13). I also saw that I had to make a right choice (see Rom. 8:6). I chose to set my mind on Him and His will for my life.

What changes did I make 10 years ago that I still practice? I get up early to study the Bible, pray and exercise. I still attend a weekly First Place meeting. For the greater part of the 10 years, I've led a First Place group and have helped others learn what I have learned. Today I am strong, energetic, confident and able to accomplish so much at home, in the church and in the community.

Recently, a friend and I started an exercise group that meets at our church four times a week. We launched this group because we wanted to participate. And when I go grocery shopping, I purchase healthy foods that are nutritious and good for us. The junk food stays at the store. My point is that it's all about choices.

Before I joined First Place, I managed my life my way and didn't like the results. After doing it God's way for 10 years, I like the results much better. The last 10 years have been the best 10 years of my life.

I lost 56 pounds in First Place, which put me 100 pounds lower than my heaviest weight. I've gained 15 to 20 pounds, but I still maintain a size and weight I like. I sleep well at night and I wake feeling rested. Body aches and pains are gone. The discipline I applied in the physical area of portion control and healthy choices has carried over to the mental and emotional areas, as I learned to control anger and stress. My relationship with God is so much more personal and intimate. My personal relationships are, too.

Two thoughts from two verses come to mind. Isaiah 55:8 reads, "For my thoughts are not your thoughts, neither are My ways your ways. . . . My ways are higher than your ways and My thoughts are higher than your thoughts." We have to be willing to be submissive and let go of doing things our way based on our thoughts. I certainly made a mess doing things my way. The second thought comes from 1 Corinthians 2:9: "No eye has seen, no ear has heard, no mind has conceived what God has prepared for those who love Him." This has proven true for me! My most rewarding and satisfying years of life have been the ones I have spent "living it" in First Place!

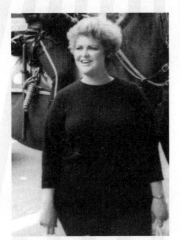

Before First Place

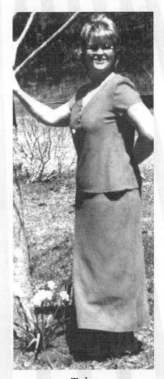

Today

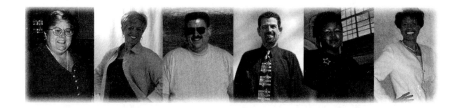

Chapter 12

VITAMINS AND MINERALS

God created you to be healthy.

DR. BEN LERNER

It seems like every time you turn around, there's new information about vitamins, minerals and other supplements. If you're like most people, you may be confused about what to do. What's true and what isn't? Let's sort through the hype.

- There are no miracle foods or supplements. Avoid anything that promises rapid results or a quick fix.
- Ignore dramatic statements that go against what most physicians, registered dietitians or national health organizations recommend.
- Stick to what you know about good nutrition, regular physical activity and a healthy lifestyle. Maintaining a well-balanced diet that includes a wide variety of foods is the best

way to obtain the nutrients you need.
  • It is wise to avoid anything that sounds too good to be true!

It's true—vitamins, minerals and phytochemicals are necessary for good health, and provide many great benefits. However, the best benefits come from food, not from supplements.

While everyone knows that it's important to eat fruits and vegetables, only 20 percent of all adults consume the minimum recommendation of five servings of fruits and vegetables each day. How many servings do you eat? Never substitute other foods for your exchanges of the fruits, vegetables and whole grains that you need to eat (see appendix on exchanges). Better yet, get lots of regular physical activity and add a few extra servings of fruits and vegetables. Studies show that eating seven or more servings a day may offer additional health benefits.

SEEKING MORE ENERGY

Vitamins and minerals *do not* supply energy—that's the job of calories from carbohydrates and fats. However, vitamins and minerals are a part of the process of changing the food you eat into the type of energy that your body can use. They're also important for many chemical reactions that take place in your body every day. The best scientific evidence suggests that your body uses vitamins and minerals best in the combinations found in food naturally.

It seems like new information about vitamins makes the news every month. You may have heard about antioxidants, homocysteine and phytochemicals. Let's look at what medical science has discovered about them.

Antioxidants
Three antioxidants are most often in the headlines: beta-carotene, vitamin E and vitamin C. Antioxidants help maintain healthy cells by protecting them against oxidation and the damaging effects of free radicals.

Free radicals are potentially damaging oxygen molecules that are produced naturally by the body. Some experts believe that environmental factors such as smoking, air pollution and other stressors increase the production of free radicals. Studies suggest that antioxidants in fruits, vegetables and other foods may help reduce the risk of heart disease, certain cancers and a variety of other health problems. Most experts feel that more studies need to be done before specific recommendations for supplementation can be made.

Antioxidants in fruits, vegetables and other foods may help reduce the risk of heart disease, certain cancers and a variety of other health problems.

Homocysteine

You may have heard about homocysteine—a protein in the blood. High levels may be associated with an increased risk of heart attack and stroke. Homocysteine levels can be influenced by what you eat. The B vitamins—folic acid, B_6 and B_{12}—help to break down homocysteine in the body. So far, there are no studies showing that taking B vitamins will lower your risk for heart attack and stroke. Everyone should follow an eating plan that has plenty of folic acid and vitamins B_6 and B_{12}. Good sources of these are citrus fruits, tomatoes, dark green leafy vegetables and fortified cereals and grain products (rice, oats and wheat flour). Eggs, fish, chicken and lean red meats are also good sources.

Phytochemicals

To protect themselves against disease, plants naturally produce these substances. These same compounds appear to have very beneficial effects on human health as well. You may have heard about phytochemicals such as isoflavones, sulphoranes, lycopene and carotenoids.

Currently there is no evidence that these chemicals can be concentrated in pill form to provide health benefits. Take your phytochemicals in the form of fruits, vegetables and whole grains.

TAKING SUPPLEMENTS

Currently none of the major health organizations such as the American Heart Association, the American Cancer Society or the American Dietetic Association recommend that healthy adults routinely take vitamin or mineral supplements for general health. There's simply not enough information on the dosages or combinations of vitamins, minerals and other nutrients that work best.

As noted above, it is best to get the vitamins, minerals and phytochemicals your body needs from the foods you eat. Supplements do not re-create what God has supplied naturally through fruits, vegetables, whole grains and other nutritious foods. Eat a variety of fruits, vegetables and whole grains each day. Balance these foods with lean meats and low-fat dairy products to get the balance and variety you need for a vitamin-packed eating plan.

What if someone is already taking vitamin and mineral supplements? There is no evidence that taking a multivitamin and mineral supplement that does not exceed the recommended daily allowances (RDAs) is associated with any harmful effects. Vitamin and mineral supplements can be an important part of an overall health plan if taking them helps you to live a healthier lifestyle—i.e., eating a healthy diet and being more physically active. In fact, standard multivitamins and mineral supplements can offer some insurance while you are actively losing weight.

However, dietary supplements are not a substitute for eating healthily! Vitamin and mineral doses higher than the RDAs should only be taken after seeking advice from your physician or a registered dietitian. For otherwise healthy people, there is only limited data suggesting advantages for taking certain vitamin or mineral supplements in excess of the RDAs.

Are dietary supplements more appropriate for certain people? Supplements may be appropriate for some people.

- People who have osteoporosis, an iron deficiency, a digestive disorder or another health condition may be treated or prevented with certain dietary supplements.
- People who follow very low-calorie eating plans or restrictive eating patterns (such as a vegetarian who consumes no meat or dairy products) may need supplements. However, we do not recommend these restrictive eating plans.
- People who can't eat certain foods may need a supplement to give the body what it needs.
- Women planning to become pregnant or who are pregnant/breast-feeding should talk to their doctor about the need for certain supplements such as folic acid and iron.

PREVENTING CANCER

There are many weight-related diseases. Cancer is just one example. Let's consider some recommendations for preventing cancer.

Consume foods high in vitamin A, especially beta-carotene. Vitamin A and beta-carotene, from which vitamin A is formed, appear to be particularly valuable in cancer prevention. About 20 studies in various parts of the world suggest an inverse association between eating foods containing vitamin A or beta-carotene and various types of human cancer, with risk reduced by 30 to 50 percent. These studies have shown that eating such foods (especially dark green and orange vegetables and various fruits) may lower the risk of cancers of the larynx, esophagus and lungs. Scientifically speaking, beta-carotene is capable of quenching singlet oxygen and peroxides that are formed in the body. Retinoids may inhibit formation of key enzymes that enhance tumor promotion. Remember, vitamin A is a fat-soluble vitamin and in excess amounts will build up to toxic levels in the body. Therefore, supplementation is unnecessary.

Consume foods high in vitamin C, vitamin E and selenium. All three of these nutrients function as or contribute to antioxidant systems in the body. These antioxidant systems help prevent the alteration of DNA that is caused by the electron-seeking free radicals. Vitamin C is found in fruits; vitamin E is found in whole grains and vegetables oils, and selenium is found in meats and whole grains.

Individuals who are 40 percent or more overweight increase their risk of colon, breast, prostate, gallbladder, ovary and uterine cancers. Women who are obese have a 44 percent greater risk, and men have a 33 percent greater risk of cancer than those of normal weight.

Include cruciferous vegetables in the diet. Cruciferous vegetables include cabbage, broccoli, brussel sprouts and cauliflower. Some studies have suggested that the consumption of these vegetables may reduce the risk of cancer, particularly of the gastrointestinal and respiratory tracts.

Don't drink alcohol or smoke tobacco. Heavy drinkers of alcohol, especially those who are also cigarette smokers, are at unusually high risk for cancers of the oral cavity, larynx, esophagus and stomach. There are approximately 40,000 studies that indicate that smoking is harmful to the body. Smoking has been determined to cause cancer in the respiratory tract (lungs). Cancer of the lungs is the leading cancer causing death.

Cut down on dietary fat (especially saturated fat) in your diet. A diet high in fat may be a factor in the development of certain cancers, particularly of the breast, colon and prostate. In addition, by restricting fatty foods, people are better able to control body weight. Most saturated fat in our diets comes from red meats, whole milk and milk products, palm oil and coconut oil. Substituting skinned chicken, turkey and fish would be helpful in reducing your consumption of red meats. Substituting low-fat milk and low-fat milk products (margarine, cheese, yogurt and the like) would also be very beneficial in reducing saturated fat. Reducing the consumption of the palm oil and coconut oil found in foods would also be helpful. Substituting olive oil (monosaturated oil) and safflower oil (polyunsaturated oil) should also be beneficial in reducing saturated fat.

Adjust your attitude. You must start making healthy decisions concerning the type of food you consume. You can't continue consuming unhealthy food just for the convenience of time or availability. The decisions you make concerning your food choices are of great importance. Every cell in your body depends on the choices you make.

The following are some healthy choices that you can make as you adopt a new attitude:

- Eat a wide variety of food each day. This will ensure the consumption of the 45 known nutrients in their proper amounts.

- Eat three well-spaced meals each day. Don't skip meals, especially breakfast.

- Control your total food intake. Don't overeat. Don't leave the table feeling stuffed. You don't have to consume everything on your plate.

Add fiber to your diet. Some studies suggest that diets high in fiber may help to reduce the risk of colon cancer. Americans now eat only 10 to 15 grams of dietary fiber a day. Populations that consume diets containing twice this amount have a lower rate of cancers of the colon and rectum. The data suggests that if a person eats 20 to 30 grams of dietary fiber each day, a 50 percent reduction in cancer of the colon and rectum is possible. In addition, foods high in fiber are a good substitute for food high in fat. "Fiber" is a term used for the plant components that are not readily digested in the human intestinal tract. Whole grain cereal products, unskinned fruits and vegetables, legumes and nuts all have dietary fiber. However, foods from animal sources (meats, milk, cheese, eggs and so on) do not have any fiber at all. Be aware that fiber supplements are not the answer. All studies to date show cancer-protective effects are associated with fiber-rich foods.

Cut down on smoked-cured meats. Smoked foods, such as hams, sausage, fish and luncheon meats, absorb some of the tars that come from incomplete combustion. These tars contain cancer-causing chemicals, similar to those of cigarette smoke. Evidence shows that salt-cured or pickled foods may increase the risk of stomach and esophageal cancer. Nitrites are used with meats to help protect against food poisoning (botulism), and to improve color and flavor. Consumption of these nitrites can lead to the formation of nitro amines, which are powerful cancer-causing chemicals. The American meat industry is working on reducing its use of nitrites.

Exercise regularly. Studies reveal that people who exercise (aerobically) at least four times per week have more interferon and interleukin—two immunity hormones—circulating in their blood than nonexercisers. These hormones stimulate the immunity system that in turn may protect against cancer. Maybe this is why physically fit children miss fewer days of school because of illness than the unfit children. Physically fit adults also miss fewer days of work than the unfit adult.

Reap the benefits. We need to practice our own preventive medicine. To believe that "it can't happen to me" is not only foolish and dangerous but also unrealistic. Yes, cancer can occur in any of us who ignorantly or willfully defy God's natural laws. We should not blame God that we don't give up these self-destructive eating habits. We know the rules and the penalties for breaking them. Cause and effect, the underlying principle of natural law, is the first fundamental belief taught in the scientific method. To ignore it leads to our destruction. Eat correctly, reap the benefits, and give honor and glory to God through your body.

—*Dr. Richard Couey*

KEITH YAWN

Hattiesburg, Mississippi

I used to have a "wait" problem: I couldn't wait until the next time I could eat. Any food would do, and the more of it there was, the better. I would eat too much at meals and then turn around and eat too much for snacks between the meals. At the same time that I was overeating, I would have told you that I was on a diet.

Actually, as far as diets go, I had tried them all. I was what I now call a Monday morning dieter. When I went to bed on Sunday nights, I would say to myself, *OK, starting tomorrow morning I'm going on a diet.* Mad at myself for my past failures, I would add, *This time I'm going to lose weight! This time it's going to be different. This time I can do it if I just try hard enough.* It would work. I would lose weight, but as soon as my willpower ran out (usually after about a week of dieting), the weight would come back—plus a few extra pounds.

I had some health problems, so there was not much doubt that I needed to lose weight. Finally, one day I had had enough. I was through trying. I was through failing. I came to the conclusion that I could not lose weight on my own—I could not do it. Just when I gave up trying on my own, the Lord stepped in and took over.

The morning after I had given up, I heard about a program held at my church. My wife had previously mentioned the First Place program to me, but this time I really thought it was for me. I heard the Lord say that this was it. This was the answer to the question I had so desperately been asking.

The following Sunday I began my new life—a life in which the Lord allows me to conquer my old cravings, create new habits and control my eating binges. Thirty-five pounds ago I endured life; now I enjoy every day. I am closer to the Lord than ever. I have more energy. I live life to the fullest. I can enjoy my kids more. The list of ways my life is now better goes on and on. To sum up my experience in First Place I would say that by myself I would never have done it, but with my Lord and Savior all things are possible.

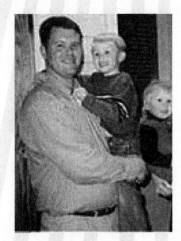

Before First Place

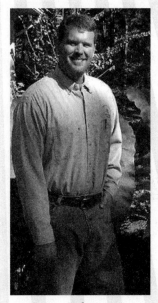

Today

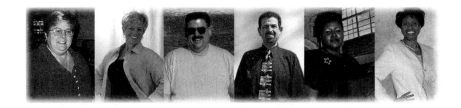

QUESTIONS AND ANSWERS ABOUT FOOD

Mom, can we go to McDonald's?

AMBER, AGE 9

We all have questions about what we can eat. In this chapter I answer a wide brushstroke of the most common queries that I have heard over the years.[1]

I love milk, but it upsets my stomach. What should I do?
A common carbohydrate disorder is lactose intolerance. If lactose is not digested by lactase in the small intestine, it then travels into the colon. Bacteria in the colon metabolize the lactose into acids and gas. About two hours after consuming milk products, the person with lactose intolerance then experiences abdominal distention and gas symptoms associated with drinking milk.

    If you have lactose intolerance, do not relinquish all milk and milk products, because these are very good sources of calcium, riboflavin, potassium and magnesium. Several options are available to those who prefer to continue using milk products. First, they should consume smaller serving sizes of milk products and take them with other foods. This usually works, probably because their digestive systems can digest some lactose, but not large loads. Second, they can eat cheese. Much lactose is lost when milk is made into cheese. Finally, they can consume yogurt. The bacteria that make yogurt can provide their own lactase activity so that lactose in yogurt essentially digests itself.

Is sugar bad for you?

Many people think it is not healthy to consume sugars. True, simple sugars by themselves have very low nutrient densities. In other words, sugary foods may supply few, if any, vitamins, minerals or proteins compared with the number of calories they supply. However, if one can afford to consume some extra calories, there is probably nothing wrong with eating sugar. Scientists estimate that sugar is mostly a problem when substituted for more nutritious foods. In that case, a person could become deficient in vitamins and other important nutrients.

In the final analysis, use of sugar should follow the safe advice given for many other food products—moderation. By regularly visiting the dentist and keeping blood sugar levels and weight under control, sugar can be enjoyed in moderation, meaning a limit of about 10 percent of total calorie intake.

Is honey better for you than sugar?

It so happens that honey, like table sugar, contains glucose and fructose. The only difference is that in table sugar they are hitched together, and in honey some of them are not. Like table sugar, honey is concentrated to the point that it contains very few impurities, even such desirable ones as vitamins and minerals. In fact, being a liquid, honey is denser than its crystalline counterpart and so contains more calories per spoon (16 calories per teaspoon for white sugar; 22 calories per teaspoon for honey).

Honey basically offers the same nutritional value as other simple sugar sources—a source of energy and little else. However, honey is not safe to use with infants because it can contain spores of the bacterium clostridium botulinum. These spores can become the bacteria that cause fatal food poisoning.

Should children follow a low-fat diet?

Although the topic is still somewhat controversial and more studies are needed, cardiologists generally agree that limiting your child's fat intake from age three onward will help reduce the odds against eventually developing coronary heart disease.

Cutting back on high-fat fast foods, like chicken fingers and fries; junk foods, like chips and cookies; and high-fat desserts is a start. Parents can start by substituting fresh fruit, raw vegetables and fruit smoothies for high fat treats.

Fast-food restaurants are beginning to substitute fruit and salads for some of the high-fat items in their kid's meals. Many school lunch programs are also trying to offer healthier selections so that children can cut down on the amount of fat they eat.

Does ice cream contain a lot of fat?

Each year, Americans consumed 15 quarts (120 scoops) for every man, woman and child. To be called ice cream, a frozen confection must contain at least 10 percent butterfat (8 percent, if it's chocolate or strawberry) and weigh at least 4.5 pounds per gallon. Ice milk, by law, needs only 2 to 7 percent butterfat, while sherbet may contain as little as 1 to 2 percent butterfat. In practical terms, these regulations mean that the average scoop of ice cream (½ cup) contains roughly 135 calories, 65 of which are fat, while ice milk has 90 calories, 25 of which are fat, and sherbet has about 135 calories, of which only 9 are fat. (The reason sherbet has as many calories as ice cream, despite the fact that it has much less fat, is that it has much more sugar and is denser.)

What is the recommended fat, carbohydrate and protein intake?

Recommendations for protein intake have changed over the years. In

2002, the Institute of Medicine released the following recommendations on how much fat, carbohydrates and protein that people should
consume:

- Adults should get 45 percent to 65 percent of their calories
  from carbohydrates, 20 percent to 35 percent from fat, and 10
  to 35 percent from protein. Acceptable ranges for children are
  similar to those for adults, except that infants and younger
  children need a slightly higher proportion of fat (25 percent to
  40 percent).
- To maintain cardiovascular health, regardless of weight, adults
  and children should exercise each day.
- Added sugars should comprise no more than 25 percent of
  total calories consumed. Added sugars are those incorporated
  into foods and beverages during production, which usually
  provide insignificant amounts of vitamins, minerals or other
  essential nutrients. Major sources include soft drinks, fruit
  drinks, pastries, candy and other sweets.
- The recommended intake for total fiber for adults 50 years and
  younger is set at 38 grams for men and 25 grams for women,
  while for men and women over 50 it is 30 and 21 grams per day,
  respectively, due to decreased food consumption.
- Using new data, the report reaffirms previously established recommended levels of protein intake, which is 0.8 grams per kilo-
  gram of body weight for adults; however recommended levels
  during pregnancy are increased.
- The report doesn't set maximum levels for saturated fat, cholesterol, or trans fatty acids, as increased risk exists at levels
  above zero, however the recommendation is to eat as little as
  possible while consuming a diet adequate in important other
  essential nutrients.
- Recommendations are made for linoleic acid (an omega-six
  fatty acid) and for alpha-linolenic acid (an omega-three fatty
  acid).[2]

How can vegetarians get protein?

The vegetarian has the same nutritional tasks as any other person: planning a diet that will deliver a variety of foods to provide all the 45 known nutrients within an energy allowance that won't cause weight gain or loss. The added challenge comes from doing so with at least one less food group.

The possibility of a protein deficiency from a vegetarian diet is remote, assuming that the vegetarian consumes enough energy. Only when fruits and certain poorly chosen vegetables define the core of the diet might protein deficiency result. Fruits provide adequate energy, but most are low in protein. A wise use of time and energy would be to obtain, prepare and eat a wide variety of foods to obtain adequate energy, protein and other nutrients. An advantage of vegetarian protein foods is that they are generally lower in fat than meats and are often higher in fiber and richer in certain vitamins and minerals as well.

I've heard that adults should not drink milk. Is that true?

Most experts recommend that adults should consume at least three servings of milk and milk products daily. Do you fear that you will consume unwanted calories? A glass of skim milk contains few calories and very little cholesterol or saturated fat. Calcium supplements can also be a good source of calcium, but they do not contain the riboflavin (B_2) and protein that milk products do.

Where are the leanest cuts of meat found on a cow?

The leanest cuts are the parts that get the most exercise when an animal moves. Since the neck, shoulders, legs and belly work more than the areas along the mid backbone, meat from the chuck (neck and shoulders), shank (lower leg), flank (belly) and round (upper back leg) tends to have more muscle and less fat than meat from the ribs, loin and sirloin, the least exercised parts.

How does body fat influence appetite?

For those who become overweight as a result of their overactive appetites, the problem may be compounded by the presence of the extra fat itself. That's because any excess fat cells the body acquires apparently fight to stay the size they are; they do not idly jiggle by, waiting to shrink into oblivion the moment someone begins to follow a weight-reducing regimen. Fat's tenacious hold on the body may have something to do with what researchers today call a person's set point—that is, a sort of internal thermostat that keeps body weight more or less constant. What the set point theory maintains, in effect, is that once weight gain has been stopped, a fat plateau has been reached and the body will do everything it can to stay at that plateau.

Some scientists think that fat cells may work to maintain the plateau, or set point, by diverting energy away from the muscles and the body's organs and into the layer of adipose tissue. Such a shift would not only allow fat cells to maintain their size but also lead to a greater appetite. Obviously, the more fat cells someone has, the worse the vicious circle of overeating to compensate for misplaced energy.

How can I control calorie intake?

The best foods to eat when trying to lose weight are those high in carbohydrates. Carbohydrates provide less than half as many calories as fat (1 gram of fat=9 calories; 1 gram of carbohydrate=4 calories). A weight-loss plan should include at least 150 grams of carbohydrate daily to prevent ketosis and reduce the risk of binging on large amounts of food, particularly sweets, because of intense hunger.

Do not reduce the fat content of a diet below 20 percent of the total calorie intake. A diet too low in fat produces very little satiety, so hunger returns very quickly after eating. A diet that contains 30 percent of its calories as fat permits a person to incorporate most commonly eaten foods into the diet. Even subtle changes in food habits can produce desired weight loss. Changing habits appropriately is the key both to losing weight and to maintaining a desirable weight.

Normally, most people need to lose fewer than 50 pounds. By consuming a lower-calorie diet, these people should be able to achieve a desirable weight within one year. Remember, it took time to gain weight. It takes time to lose it.

What constitutes a good weight-loss diet?

A good weight-loss diet should include management of three types of activities: controlling calorie intake, changing problem food-choice habits and increasing physical activity. A diet that focuses on just eating fewer calories is not complete enough to be successful. Specifically, look for the following characteristics:

1. The diet should include all of the 45 known nutrients in their proper amounts.
2. Rapid weight loss should be discouraged. A slow and steady weight loss should be stressed. A loss of 1 to 2 pounds per week of fat storage would be ideal.
3. The diet should not have rigid rituals, such as only eating fruit in the morning or not eating meat after milk products.
4. The diet should contain at least 1,200 calories per day. A lower calorie-consumption level could cause the body to convert protein (lean body tissue) to glucose, because of insufficient carbohydrate in the diet. In addition, it is almost impossible to consume enough iron, especially for young women, if the diet calls for fewer calories than 1,500 per day. If the diet calls for fewer calories than this per day, it should recommend either fortified foods (for example, breakfast cereals) or a balanced vitamin and mineral supplement to supply iron.
5. Remember, no magical food can speed weight loss. If a diet suggests one—for example, tofu, garlic or grapefruit)—find another diet.
6. The diet should emphasize behavior modification to overcome bad eating habits. The diet should stress ways to make lifestyle changes that can reshape poor eating habits, along with ways to maintain weight maintenance so as to thwart further weight gain.
7. The diet should not only stress good eating practices but also emphasize regular physical activity, stress reduction and other healthy changes in lifestyle.

8. A sound weight-loss diet should allow you to participate in social activities, such as eating at a restaurant or at a party.

9. A diet should encourage the dieter to see a physician for a good physical checkup, especially if the dieter has previous health problems, such as heart disease or diabetes.

Notes

1. Much of the information in this chapter was provided by Dr. Richard Couey, professor of health sciences, Baylor University, Waco, Texas, and is used by permission.

2. "Dietary Reference Intakes for Energy, Carbohydrate, Fiber, Fat, Fatty Acids, Cholesterol, Protein, and Amino Acids," *Institute of Medicine of the National Academies,* September 5, 2002. http://www.iom.edu/report.asp?id=4340 (accessed October 28, 2004).

CAROL PEAVY

Jena, Louisiana

Little did I know what God had in store for me when I joined First Place in January 1996. At that point in my life, I was only looking to lose some weight.

After having tried various diets and even diet pills for many years with no permanent results to show for all of the effort, a friend told me about a First Place group which was meeting at a local church. I knew nothing about the program, but I was desperate. So with nothing to lose but weight, I decided to give it a try.

During the first 13-week session, I lost 18 pounds, but I still wasn't willing to participate in leading prayer or Bible study at the meetings. After a few months I no longer needed my medicine for high blood pressure. By the time I finished the next two sessions (39 weeks after I began), I had lost a total of 40 pounds! But more important than the weight loss was the fact that I began stepping out for the Lord. I began studying my Bible, meeting with the Lord in a quiet time, praying and exercising.

Without First Place I would not be where I am today—healthier, a committed exerciser, growing in the Lord and soaring to new levels with Him every day.

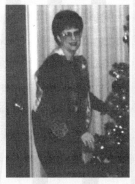

Before First Place

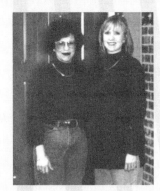

Today

Part IV

THE FITNESS
CONNECTION

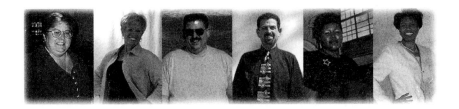

Chapter 14

THE IMPORTANCE OF BEING FIT

Better health is an individual responsibility and an important national goal.

PRESIDENT GEORGE W. BUSH

Weight gain and obesity are often viewed as problems of eating too much. While this is part of the problem, obesity is just as likely to result from too little physical activity. Many experts feel that the alarming increase in being overweight and obese is a result of the sedentary lifestyles of most Americans. Today nearly 25 percent of Americans are completely sedentary, and up to 60 percent do not get enough physical activity to benefit their health. Increasing physical activity—energy expenditure—is as important to weight control as decreasing calorie intake.

An important study published in the *American Journal of Clinical Nutrition* surveyed nearly 800 men and women from the National Weight Control Registry who maintained an average weight loss of more than 60 pounds for over 5 years. In this survey, 90 percent of the participants reported regular physical activity as a part of their program. Other studies have reported similar findings.

A series of studies reported by researchers from the Cooper Institute for Aerobics Research in Dallas, Texas, reveal that death rates from all causes are much lower in obese men with a moderate to high level of physical fitness than in normal-weight men with low physical fitness. These important studies confirm that a lifestyle of physical activity and healthy eating is more important than the number on the scale. In other words, as the researchers from this study reported: It's better to be fit and fat than lean and sedentary.

FITNESS BENEFITS

What are the benefits of being fit? You will find that fitness

- helps the body burn fat and protects against the muscle loss associated with low-calorie eating plans;
- helps the body maintain or increase its metabolic rate;
- may help suppress appetite;
- allows for weight loss on a higher calorie eating plan, which helps the body get all the nutrients it needs;
- improves mood and self-esteem;
- results in important health benefits such as lower blood pressure, improved cholesterol levels and increased fitness;
- promotes long-term weight maintenance.

Obstacles

No time, no fun and *bo-or-or-ring!* These are common reasons that people give for not making physical activity a lifetime habit. Yet experts are making it harder and harder to come up with good excuses. The latest recommendations tell us that exercise doesn't have to be hard to be beneficial. Gone are the days when you had to exercise for at least 30 minutes at a certain heart rate to get the health and fitness benefits of aerobic exercise.

What's the exercise prescription for today? Something is better than nothing, and more is better than something.

The latest recommendations from groups such as the American Heart Association and the American College of Sports Medicine call for at least 30 minutes of moderate physical activity on as many days of the week as possible. The latest twist on this new recommendation is that the activity doesn't have to be done all at one time. Shorter amounts accumulated over the course of a day appear to offer the same health benefits as the more traditional 30 continuous minutes of exercise.

Solutions

Shorter workouts are easier to start and to stick with. It's easy to get burned out on exercise by doing too much too soon. Start slow and work your way up to longer sessions as your physical activity becomes a habit.

You may also be a person who just doesn't have 30 to 60 minutes to give at one time. Shorter workouts are easier to fit into your schedule and will help fight boredom by allowing more variety in your routine. They're also great for regular exercisers who occasionally miss or are unable to do their usual routine. When you miss or know you are going to miss a session, just slip in one or two of these shorter workouts wherever and whenever you can.

Are lack of time, lack of enjoyment and boredom among the reasons you have a hard time making exercise a part of your life? Whether you're a regular exerciser or just getting started, consider some of the following ideas for fitting 10-minute walking workouts into your day:

- Walking can be done anywhere, anytime. Think about times in your typical day when you can fit in a short, brisk walk.
- Get up 10 minutes earlier and fit in a quick walk before starting your day.
- Walk each day. You can pray or meditate while you walk.

- Take 10-minute walking breaks at work.
- Arrive to work 10 minutes early and walk or climb the stairs.
- Take a 10-minute walk around the mall before stopping to shop.
- Walk your dog for 10 minutes.
- Take the entire family out for a 10-minute walk before or after meals.
- Walk around the house during commercials or between shows—you'll easily get in 10 minutes.

Walking is not your only choice for exercise. Here are some other creative ideas:

- Pick up the pace when you're doing household chores. Ten minutes of vacuuming, washing the car or working in the yard add up over the course of a day. To get the benefit, however, you have to push the pace a bit. Turn on your favorite music to help keep you moving.
- Buy an exercise video and pop it in for 10 minutes.
- Do you have exercise equipment that's collecting dust? Pull it out and try a 10-minute routine instead of feeling like you have to stay on for 30 minutes or longer.
- Rather than just watching your kids play, spend 10 minutes playing with them: Shoot baskets, throw a ball or Frisbee, or kick a soccer ball.
- Take 10-minute breaks at work and do calisthenics, strength training or stretching exercises.

Choose a few activities that you enjoy and can do for approximately 10 minutes at a time. Be creative—don't limit yourself to the traditional exercises. Whatever you choose to do, try to make it fun. Remember, the *e* in "exercise" is for *enjoyment!*

Once you've chosen a few activities, find some times you can fit them into your day. Think about times in your day when you can be more active, such as when you are watching television, shopping, working around the house or taking a break. Heed the public service announcement that has aired on the radio that says, "Take the stairs rather than elevator!"

Outdoor Exercises

One of the best ways to get active is to get out and enjoy God's beautiful creation. There are many enjoyable and beneficial activities you can do outdoors, such as walking, hiking, bicycling, swimming and participating in other recreational sports. However, when it comes to exercising outdoors, there are several things you can do to increase the enjoyment and safety of the activities you choose. It's important to consider weather, clothing, equipment and environment when exercising outdoors. Also, some activities such as downhill skiing, in-line skating and bicycling are more risky and require more precautions for safety. Choose activities you enjoy, but *take it slow and play it smart!*

When exercising outdoors, there are several things you need to keep in mind to prevent injury or illness. A good pair of shoes is the most important piece of equipment for exercising outdoors. Here are some tips for selecting a pair of exercise shoes.

- The best shoe is the one that fits your foot well; it's not necessarily the most expensive. Try on several pairs before buying. Does the shoe feel natural when you walk? Keep trying until you find one that feels right!
- Make sure the shoe supports your arch and has plenty of room for your toes; allow for a thumb's width between your toes and the end of the shoe. Keep your toenails trimmed!
- For walking or jogging, choose a flexible shoe with good cushioning. Don't go hiking in tennis shoes; wear the appropriate boot or shoe.
- For court and field sports, consider a high-top shoe to protect your ankles.
- Wear cotton or nylon athletic socks. It's not necessary to wear a double layer of socks.

When deciding what clothing to wear, consider the weather and light conditions.

- Whether exercising in the heat or cold, always wear clothing that can be layered and easily removed or put back on, as your body temperature changes.
- Check with a local sports store for the best clothing and protective gear for your activity.
- At dusk or at night, wear reflective and light-colored clothing, and carry a flashlight.
- Consider carrying a small backpack or fanny pack to store extra clothing.
- When exercising in the heat, avoid clothing that does not ventilate well, such as rubberized suits or sweat suits. Wearing such clothing is a dangerous practice that can lead to dehydration and heat stroke!

Extreme temperatures affect how your body responds to exercise. High temperatures and humidity or cold temperatures and wind place additional stress on your body. Check the weather forecast before heading outdoors. *Always decrease your intensity level and take it slow when it's very hot or cold!*

Here are some tips for beating the heat:

- It's a hot day when the temperature is above 85 degrees Fahrenheit or when the temperature plus the humidity is greater than 130 (i.e., 80 degrees plus 55 percent humidity equals 135).
- It takes 10 to 14 days to adapt to the heat. If you're exercising in hot conditions, cut your intensity and duration in half and gradually increase your activity as your body adapts to the heat.
- Drink water before, during and after exercise. Drink at least five to eight ounces of cool water 15 minutes before and then every 15 to 20 minutes during exercise.

- On really hot days, exercise during the coolest part of the day or exercise indoors.
- Wear lightweight, loose-fitting clothes, a hat and sunscreen to protect you from the sun. If you wear a hat, make sure it allows for ventilation.

Here are some tips to beat the cold:

- Don't just rely on the thermometer; the wind-chill factor greatly increases the risk of exercising in the cold.
- Dress warmly and in layers that can be easily removed. Several layers warm better than one heavy jacket. Because physical activity quickly generates body heat, it's important to be able to remove layers as your body heats up.
- Wool and synthetic fabrics are good choices because they whisk moisture away from your body. Wear an outer layer that keeps out the wind and moisture.
- Much of your body's heat can be lost through your head and neck, so wear a hat and scarf. Don't forget to protect your hands, too.
- Watch out for slick surfaces caused by rain and snow.
- It's just as important to drink water in the cold as it is in the heat.
- When exercising in the cold, stay close to home or another shelter.

STRETCHING FOR FLEXIBILITY

Stretching is a simple and relaxing activity that offers a variety of important health and fitness benefits. A regular program of stretching exercises gives you increased flexibility in your muscles and joints, which helps you feel more relaxed, prevents injury and improves your ease of movement. Stretching also prevents the loss of flexibility and the pain and stiffness that make doing even simple activities difficult later in life. Unfortunately, flexibility is the most often overlooked part of an activity program.

Are you flexible enough?

- Are your muscles and joints sore and stiff after yard work, exercise or recreational activities?
- Are you sore and stiff when you wake up in the morning?
- Do you feel less agile and flexible than you did a few years ago?
- Does your range of motion seem limited when doing certain activities?

Altitude increases the stress of physical activity. It's harder for your body to take in oxygen above 5,000 feet. This means that your heart, lungs and muscles have to work harder. Symptoms of altitude sickness include lightheadedness, dizziness, nausea and unusual shortness of breath. Give yourself a couple of days to get used to the higher elevation and cut back the intensity of your activities.

—Dr. Jody Wilkinson

If you answered yes to any of these questions, you'll probably benefit from a program of regular stretching. Remember that flexibility is important for overall health and well-being, too.

Stretching should be done as part of your warm-up before and your cooldown after physical activity. You may also want to do a routine program of stretching several times each week. In fact, stretching can be done any time.

Guidelines for Safe Stretching

The following are some guidelines to stretch safely:

- Before stretching, warm up your body with 3 to 5 minutes of light activity.
- All stretches should be performed slowly and smoothly. Never bounce or jerk.

- Focus your mind on the muscles and joints you're stretching and keep your body relaxed.
- Stretch to the point that you feel mild muscle tension. Don't stretch to the point of pain! Overstretching will do more harm than good.
- Hold each stretch for 15 to 20 seconds. Relax and breathe easily during each stretch. Never hold your breath.
- Avoid stretches that cause you to arch your back or neck backward or that put stress on your knees.
- Don't do any stretch that could cause you to lose your balance and fall.
- Never compare yourself with others. Flexibility is not about how far you can stretch; it's about loosening and relaxing the muscles and joints.

Whole-Body Stretches

The following exercises are basic stretches for the major muscles and joints. Spend more time on your stiffest areas, but try to do all these stretches several times each week. You can do all the stretches at one time or do different stretches at different times of the day. The best way is to start with your neck and work your way down. Repeat each of the following stretches two to three times. Remember to relax, go slow and enjoy the time you spend stretching. Stretching is a great time to pray and meditate on Scripture.

Neck. These neck exercises can be done sitting or standing.

- While looking straight ahead, tilt your head to the side as though you're trying to touch your ear to your shoulder. Hold the stretch for a few seconds; then repeat the movement to the other side.
- Next, try to touch your chin to your chest. Go down only as far as is comfortable, hold for a few seconds and take a deep breath. Return to the starting position.

Shoulders and arms. The following shoulder and arm exercises can be done sitting or standing.

- Reach up and over your head with one or both arms, as if trying to touch the ceiling. Bend slightly to each side. Repeat with the other arm.
- Next, reach forward with one arm and then stretch it across your chest toward the opposite shoulder. Increase the stretch by pulling with the opposite arm. Repeat with the other arm.
- Starting with your arms at your side, shrug your shoulders by bringing them up toward your ears. Lower your shoulders while stretching them backward, pulling the shoulder blades together. Return to the starting position with your arms at your sides.
- Hold your arms straight out to the side. Make wide circles with your arms, both forward and backward, by turning them at the shoulder. Make circles with your wrists, too.

Trunk and sides. With your arms at your side and you feet at least shoulder width apart, bend toward one side while sliding your arm down the side of your hip and leg. Stretch only as far as is comfortable and watch your balance. Keep your back and neck straight while doing this stretch. Repeat, this time stretching toward the other side.

Lower back. The following exercises will aid in the flexibility of your lower back.

- While sitting in a chair with your knees bent, bend forward from the waist and slide your hands down your legs toward your toes. Bend down only as far as is comfortable. Hold the stretch for a few seconds and rise back up slowly.
- Lie on your back with your knees bent and feet flat on the ground. Use your hands to pull one knee up toward the chest, while keeping your leg bent. As you pull up, press your back gently toward the floor. Keep the opposite leg bent at a 90-degree

angle and your foot flat on the floor. Hold the stretch for a few seconds. Repeat with the other leg.

· Lie with your knees bent at a 90-degree angle and feet flat on the floor. Press the small of your back toward the floor while tightening your stomach muscles. Hold the stretch for a few seconds.

· Kneel on your hands and knees and relax your neck. Arch your back up like a cat, feeling the stretch across your back. Hold for a few seconds. Repeat.

Legs and ankles. These exercises will help aid in the flexibility of your legs and ankles.

· Sit on the floor. With your legs extended and your knees slightly bent, stretch forward at the waist and try to touch your toes. You don't have to touch your toes—just bend forward until you feel a stretch in the back of your legs. Keep your head and back as straight as possible and breathe easily.

· Standing, face a wall with your arms extended straight out in front of you. Move one foot forward and leave the other foot back one to two feet. Keeping the heel of your back foot on the ground and toes pointing forward, lean your body toward the wall until you feel a mild stretch in your calf and heel. Hold the stretch for a few seconds. Repeat the stretch by changing the position of your feet.

· To loosen up your ankle muscles, stand or sit and draw an imaginary circle with your foot by turning your foot at the ankle. Do circles in both directions. Repeat several times with each foot.

SPORTS AND RECREATIONAL ACTIVITIES

There are many different ways to fit physical activity into your lifestyle.

The first step is to find activities you enjoy. Then you need to get out there and do them on a regular basis. Sports and recreational activities can be a great way to fit in physical activity. Check out the following benefits:

- They strengthen muscles, burn calories and reduce stress just as well as other types of exercise.
- They provide opportunities to enjoy your health and fitness. Playing and having fun helps you stay young and keeps you motivated.
- They allow you to spend time with family and friends and meet new people, too! Remember, relationships are just as important to your overall health and well-being as exercise and good nutrition.
- The competitive nature of some sports can inspire you to set fitness goals and stay motivated. Setting a goal such as finishing a 10 kilometer race or playing in a tennis league can make your workouts more meaningful.

No matter what your skill, coordination or fitness level, you can find activities to enjoy. Find one or two sports or recreational activities you enjoy, and fit them into your fitness routine one to three times each week. Consider the following list of possibilities:

Badminton	Golf	Skiing	Tennis
Basketball	Hiking	Soccer	Volleyball
Bike rallies	Racquetball	Softball	
Fun runs/walks	Skating	Squash	

Individual Sports and Activities

- **Fun Runs/Walks.** Many people enjoy participating in local fun runs or walks. These community events offer challenge and camaraderie. Most people don't run to compete with others; their goal is to finish the race and feel good about their accomplishment. Training for a local event is a great way to keep you motivated and add variety to your exercise routine. Joining a walking or running group is a great way to meet other people with similar interests.

- **Bike Rallies.** If you enjoy bicycling, you might want to train for a bike rally. Bike rallies are generally anywhere from 25 to 100 miles long. Choose your distance and start training. Training for a rally is a great motivator. Participating in a rally provides a great source of accomplishment and is a fun way to meet other people. Well-organized rides attract thousands of riders of all fitness levels and create a fun and exciting environment. Most cities also have bicycle clubs that get together on the weekends for longer rides and fellowship. *Never do a longer event, whether walking, running or cycling, without proper training.*

- **Skating.** There are several ways to skate these days. The two most popular ways are in-line skating (i.e., Rollerblading) and ice-skating. Actually, in-line skating is one of the fastest growing recreational activities in this country. Skating is a great aerobic exercise and a good way to burn calories. Skating does take a little more skill than walking, jogging or bicycling, and the risk of injury is much higher. Before making the investment, rent a pair of skates and take formal lessons. When in-line skating, wear wrist guards, protective padding and a helmet.

- **Skiing.** Many people have the opportunity to go downhill skiing one or more times each year. The annual ski trip can be a great motivator to keep yourself in shape. To ski enjoyably and safely you need a moderate to high level of cardiovascular endurance, muscular fitness, flexibility, balance and coordination. Spend at least two or three months getting yourself in condition to go skiing. The risk of injury during skiing is very high, and the injuries can be severe: broken bones and torn ligaments. High altitude and cold temperatures are also important safety considerations.

- **Golf.** This popular sport provides a great opportunity to enjoy the outdoors. Golf is more of a game of skill than it is of physical fitness. However, by walking and carrying your own clubs, golf can count toward your weekly physical activity goal. Physical fitness can improve your game. To be successful in golf, focus on three components of fitness: strength/power, flexibility and cardiovascular endurance. Cardiovascular endurance is essential to help keep your energy up during a long round of golf. Flexibility exercises increase your range of motion and prevent injury. Muscular fitness can improve the power and speed of your swing.

Racquet Sports

Racquet sports, such as tennis, racquetball and squash, are popular and can be played as singles or doubles. All of them offer a moderate to vigorous workout, depending on the intensity you put into it. Playing singles usually requires more effort and burns more calories. In addition to enjoying health and fitness benefits, you will also develop balance, agility and coordination. The more fit you are, the better you'll play. Develop a regular fitness routine to help improve your game and lower your risk of injury. You need cardiovascular endurance, flexibility and strength to play your best.

For equipment all you need to play is a good pair of shoes, a racquet (or just your hand for handball), a partner and a court. Shoes are probably your most important piece of equipment. You'll need a good court shoe with adequate cushioning. You'll also need good heel and ankle support because these sports have a lot of side-to-side movement. Many of the sports require protective eyewear. Check with a YMCA, local fitness club or recreation center to sign up for lessons, or find a local racquet club to help you improve your game and meet other people.

Team Sports

Team sports such as basketball, softball, volleyball and soccer have both fitness and social benefits. These sports can be light, moderate or vigorous in intensity, depending on the sport and how hard you play.

Regardless of the intensity, including team sports in your fitness program can offer a variety of benefits. Low-intensity sports, such as softball and volleyball, are great outlets for competition and fellowship. Regardless of the sport you choose, the more fit you are, the better you'll play. You need cardiovascular endurance, muscular fitness and flexibility to play your best.

Be careful if you play team sports only sporadically. It's easy to let the competitive drive take over and overexert yourself—the weekend-warrior syndrome. Some sports can take a greater toll on your body, especially as you grow older. Make sure you wear the appropriate shoes and protective gear. As you would for any exercise, spend some time warming up with light activity and stretching before playing. Cool down gradually after playing vigorous sports, such as basketball or soccer.

Thirty minutes of moderate physical activity on 5 or more days a week reduces the risk of developing or dying from the following health conditions:

- Heart disease
- High blood pressure
- Colon cancer
- Type 2 diabetes

Building physical activity into your daily routine can help add years to your life and can make your older years a high quality time of life.

—Lynn C. Swann, chairman, President's Council on Physical Fitness and Sports

BOB LENTO

Spokane, Washington

I am 37 years old and I have lost 45 pounds on the First Place program. One Friday I prayed to the Lord, telling Him that I didn't feel great about myself. I needed to lose weight, but I needed the proper vehicle to make it happen. I needed direction. The next day, my wife and I stepped into our local Christian bookstore, and the First Place program display was there, staring us in the face. It was an answer to my prayer.

In the past, I had tried other programs, especially the expensive ones that include the food, thus eliminating the guesswork. I lost weight, but I was never able to keep it off. I never learned the nutritional value of various foods, and I never brought Bible study, prayer, exercise or accountability into the process.

Now I am back in the Word of God on a daily basis, I have renewed my prayer life and I am building up my level of confidence. I was surprised by how much I learned about the food I eat, including how to count calories and how to calculate food exchanges. What I learned will enable me to keep the weight off.

The process was a bit tedious, especially at first. After all, it required a serious commitment of my time and effort, but I had to be serious about making a change in my eating habits, as well as in my spiritual life, if I wanted to see a difference.

There are no First Place groups in our area, so my wife and I became our own group and we had a "meeting" with each other once a week in our home. This had the added benefit of opening wider the doors of communication in our marriage. I am now on maintenance (maintaining my weight at a lower level), and I am doing great! I'm feeling as though my whole outlook on the way I eat, as well as life in general, has been renewed.

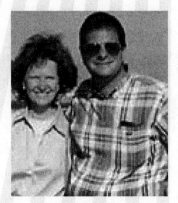

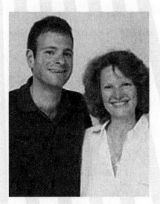

Before First Place   *Today*

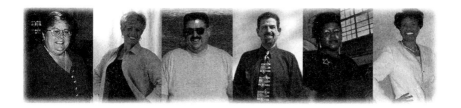

Chapter 15

SMART WORKOUT CHOICES

I would rather exercise than read a newspaper.

KIM ALEXIS

"I do not have time to exercise." "I do not have a treadmill at home." "I do not like running at the park where people might see me." "It is too expensive to buy those special shoes." There are as many excuses to not exercise as there are people who need to exercise, but if you are serious about weight loss and healthy living, you must find the willpower to take that first step.

FITNESS AT HOME

Many people find it easiest to join a gym that offers a variety of workout equipment and classes. However, you don't have to join a fitness center to get the benefits of exercise. There are many great ways to fit physical activity into your life. Choose activities that you enjoy and can fit into your lifestyle. With a little planning, you can get all the physical activity you need in the comfort and convenience of your own home.

Advantages

- **Convenience**—No travel time and no special hours are required, and you don't have to worry about what to wear.
- **Privacy**—You can work out in the comfort of your own home and at your own speed, with no overcrowding.
- **Cost**—Depending on what activity and equipment you choose, exercising at home can be very economical.

Disadvantages

- **Less Variety**—A fitness center offers a greater variety of exercise and equipment options.
- **Self-Discipline**—Some people have a hard time motivating themselves to work out alone.
- **Distractions**—The television, telephone, spouse, kids and household chores may compete for your time and attention.
- **Cost**—Some fitness equipment may cost as much or more than a club membership.

There is no best exercise or piece of exercise equipment. The best one is the one that is right for you. Any activity that requires you to use your muscles or causes you to breathe a little harder is good for your body. Walking, jogging, bicycling, dancing and strength training are good examples. Choose the one you like best and do it regularly.

HOME EXERCISE EQUIPMENT

Don't just buy a piece of exercise equipment because you think it will be good for you. Here are some things to ask yourself before you buy:

- What do I enjoy doing?
- Will I really enjoy working out at home? Why?
- Will I use the equipment regularly? Will I quickly get bored with it? (Far too common is the exercise machine that becomes an expensive clothes rack or ends up in a garage sale or thrift shop!)
- Have I used or bought home-exercise equipment before? What did I like about it? What did I dislike about it?
- Do I have a convenient place to put it?
- How much can I afford to spend? (Set a budget before you go shopping.)

When shopping for exercise equipment, look for something that gives you the feel of the activity you enjoy. You need to test equipment before you buy it. Does it seem to be well made? Does it feel solid and durable? Give the equipment a good test ride—five minutes is not enough!

All of the following types of exercise equipment are good choices:

- Treadmills
- Stair-climbers
- Skiing machines
- Rowers
- Stationary or regular bicycles
- Strength equipment
- Elastic exercise bands
- Jump ropes
- Aerobic or step videos
- Rollerblades or skates

Treadmills

Treadmills allow you to walk or jog no matter the season and no matter the weather.

- You'll need plenty of room—both in length and width—to comfortably walk or jog.

- The walking or jogging surface should be stable and provide good shock absorption (i.e., doesn't bounce or rock back and forth).
- Choose a machine with handrails for balance and a control panel that is easy to reach and use. It's best if you can adjust the speed and elevation while exercising.
- Strong motors (1¼ to 1¾ horsepower) make for a quieter and longer-lasting treadmill.

Stair-Climbing Machines

Another stationary piece, stair-climbers can be placed in the corner of a room and are relatively low impact.

- Choose a sturdy machine with good stability.
- Look for independent steps that have a smooth motion; chain or cable systems are generally smoother than hydraulic (air-powered) systems.
- It should allow for variable resistance (i.e., you set the tension, or workload).
- Make sure it is equipped with comfortable handrails.

Cross-Country Skiing Machines and Rowing Machines

A variety of stationary machines that simulate outdoor activities provide variable levels of resistance.

- Look for a machine that works both the upper and lower body.
- Look for stability; the machine shouldn't rock back and forth.
- The machine should provide smooth sliding motion of skis, with seat and arm pulleys.
- Make sure it allows for variable resistance (i.e., you set the tension, or workload).

Stationary Bikes

Stationary bikes are low impact and take up very little space in your home.

- Choose a bike with a smooth pedaling motion.
- Make sure that you're comfortable with the pedaling resistance and that it's easily adjusted.
- A comfortable, adjustable-tilt seat is a must. If bicycle seats are typically uncomfortable for you, look for a recumbent bike, which allows you to sit in a padded chair with your legs extended in front of you.
- Some bikes have arm levers that allow you to work your upper body, too.

Weights

Weights are traditional workout equipment. They strengthen muscles and increase bone density.

BEFORE YOU MAKE A PURCHASE

- If you know someone with home exercise equipment, ask to try it.
- Analyze your workout room. The area you plan to exercise in should be spacious and pleasant. It also needs to be well lit and have adequate ventilation. If you like to read or watch television while using your exercise equipment, make certain you have enough room to do so.
- Wear your workout gear when shopping so that you can test the actual equipment you will buy.
- Buy from a knowledgeable retailer. Discuss warranties, installation, maintenance and service plans.
- Check out the option of purchasing used equipment.

—Dr. Jody Wilkinson

- **Complex Systems**—Multistation resistance machines certainly have their place, but they are not affordable or practical for everyone.
- **Simple Systems**—You can get all the strength training you need with handheld weights, elastic exercise bands, dumbbells and an exercise mat or bench.

THE FITNESS CENTER

Are you looking for the best way to fit physical activity into your life? There is no *one* best way. The best way is the one that works for you. Joining a fitness center can be a great choice for some people. Fitness centers offer a wide selection of equipment and activities to help you achieve and maintain a physically active lifestyle and all the benefits that go along with it. They also provide a safe and comfortable environment in all kinds of weather, almost any time of the day.

Is joining a fitness center the right option for you? You have several options when it comes to fitting physical activity into your life. You can purchase home exercise equipment, exercise outdoors, walk in the mall or fit *lifestyle* physical activities into your daily routine (i.e., taking the

QUESTIONS TO ASK BEFORE JOINING

- **Does the club have high-pressure sales techniques?** You need to have time to think about your decision and review the contract and terms of membership. If you feel pressured, that club is probably not for you!

- **Does the center offer only (or pressure you to sign) long-term contracts (i.e., longer than one year)?** You may prefer a monthly membership at first to see if the fitness center is right for you.

- **Are the membership options and contracts hard to understand?** Contracts should be easy to understand, and options should be easy to choose from.

- **Does the fitness center representative ask you about your health and medical history?** Knowing your history is important for designing a fitness program that is right for you.

- **Does the fitness center appear to be understaffed?** You should have readily available help when you need it while working out.

—*Dr. Jody Wilkinson*

stairs instead of the elevator, working in your yard and so on). The most important thing is to choose activities that you enjoy and that fit into your lifestyle. Before joining a fitness center, ask yourself the following questions:

- Have I been a member of a fitness center before?
- If I have been a member before, did I enjoy and use the fitness center regularly?
- Can I afford all the fees (initiation, membership and classes)?
- Is there a fitness center close to my home or work?
- Do I have the time to use a fitness center regularly?
- Do I enjoy working out with others?
- Do I enjoy having a wide variety of exercise options from which to choose?
- Will I benefit from having an expert staff of fitness professionals to help me choose and maintain an effective, safe physical-activity program?
- Will joining a fitness center provide the motivation and inspiration I need to get and stay active?
- What specific benefits (i.e., equipment, group classes, supervision or amenities) am I looking for from a fitness center?

How do you choose a fitness center that's right for you? When selecting a fitness center, there are several important things to consider.

- **Is it convenient?** Studies show that you are more likely to use a center if it's within 10 to 12 minutes of your home or workplace. Remember, lack of time and inconvenient location are two common reasons people give for dropping out of a fitness program!
- **Does it provide a safe, friendly and comfortable environment?** Ask the club to allow you to work out for several days before joining—many clubs will. This helps you know whether you are comfortable in the club and it enables you to become familiar with the equipment, staff and other members. If a club

TIPS FOR GETTING THE MOST OUT OF A FITNESS CENTER

• Ask the staff to give you an orientation to the center and the equipment. Staff should always be available to answer your questions and help you use the equipment safely and effectively.

• Choose a workout time that's convenient for you. Schedule your exercise time just as you would any other important appointment.

• Choose activities and equipment you enjoy.

• Set specific goals for health and physical activity to keep you motivated.

• Get a loved one, coworker or friend to join you. The support of a buddy often keeps you on track.

• If necessary, ask for help around the house or at work so that you can fit in your workout.

—Dr. Jody Wilkinson

won't allow you a trial period, look elsewhere!

· **Is the staff trained and certified in exercise instruction and counseling?** Among the top certifications are the American College of Sports Medicine, the American Counsel on Exercise, the National Strength and Conditioning Association and the Cooper Institute.

· **Does it offer classes for all levels of fitness and skill?** Make sure the club has classes at your level at times convenient for you.

· **Does the center have a wide selection of exercise equipment?** Is the equipment clean and in good working order? Check for "out of order" signs. Check the size of the crowd at the time you will be using the facility and the availability of the equipment you'll want to use.

· **What extra features are you looking for?** Do you want a swimming pool, racquet courts, locker rooms, private showers, massage services, steam rooms, hot tubs or cafeteria?

· **How much are you willing to spend on a membership?** Do you want to pay monthly or annually?

· **What special programs and services does the club offer?** Are child care, educational programs, nutritional counseling, personal training and so on available? Are these important to you?

JESSICA MYERS

New Holland, Pennsylvania

I was obese for most of my childhood and all of my adult life. In March 2003, during a time of personal crisis, I was faced with the reality that at 312 pounds, I was putting myself at risk for some serious health problems. I also realized that, if I stayed at this weight, I might not be around to take care of my daughter—there are not many 70-year-old women who weigh as much as I did! Most important, I was not being a good steward of the body that God has given me.

> Do you not know that your body is a temple of the Holy Spirit, who is in you, whom you have received from God? You are not your own; you were bought at a price. Therefore, honor God with your body (1 Cor. 6:19-20).

As a Christian, I knew that by not taking care of my body, I was sinning, because I was not able to be all that I could be for God. I began to pray for direction. We all know how to lose weight—it is just a matter of making up our mind to do it. Eating right and exercising are the keys to success. When we are done looking for the quick fix and the easy way to accomplish our goal, we must decide either to change or to continue in the misery of disobedience.

I began researching the First Place program online and read the First Place book *Health 4 Life*. As a result, I started making small changes, such as eliminating soda and adding water to my daily diet. I began the full program on my own (as opposed to being in a group) on June 27, 2003. I also joined a gym that day. Step by step, I went through the First Place program by myself until I was able to join a group in September. I had already lost 33 pounds when I met the sweet ladies of Grace Baptist Church in Lancaster, Pennsylvania. Being part of a group makes a huge difference in motivation and it helps with success. It has been an amazing year. Time has seemed to fly by and I have had consistent success. I have truly been changed from the inside out. Although I have at times given in to temptation, I have never had a moment that I wanted to throw in the towel. That is miraculous!

To date, I have lost a total of 102 pounds! I can hardly believe it. I love telling people how I've done it—God gets all the glory. Although I am rejoicing in my physical appearance, in my higher energy level and in my nearness to God, I am eager to keep moving toward my goal of losing a total of 150 pounds. Now, I have only 48 more to go.

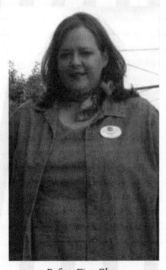 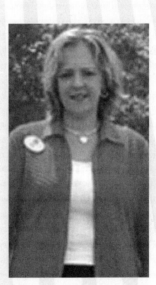

Before First Place   *Today*

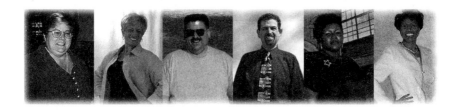

QUESTIONS AND ANSWERS ABOUT FITNESS

In order for me to be a good wife, and a good mother, and to minister to the people God puts in my path, I really need to take care of myself.

STORMIE OMARTIAN

Entire books have been written about physical fitness. In this chapter I answer some of the most common questions I have heard from people who want to lose weight and live healthy lives. Please keep in mind that no two experts will agree on exact fitness regimens—which is good, because no two people are the same. I have tapped a wide array of resources to give you a framework from which to start in each of the key areas.[1]

What is physical fitness?
Basically, fitness means being in good physical condition and being able to function at one's best level. It is the capability of the heart, blood,

lungs and muscles to function at optimal efficiency—the health needed for the most enthusiastic and pleasurable participation in daily life.

What are the components of fitness?

Exercise physiologists have divided the 10 components of fitness into two categories: health related and skill related. The health-related components are those that best improve the physiological systems of the body, whereas the skill-related components are those essential for performance in games and sports.

What is cardiovascular-respiratory fitness?

Cardiovascular-respiratory (CVR) fitness is the most important health-related component in the fitness area. As its name implies, CVR fitness means becoming fit in the heart, blood, blood vessels and lungs. Obtaining fitness in these areas reduces the probability of acquiring cardiovascular diseases such as heart attacks and strokes. These circulatory diseases are the leading causes of death among the adult population of most industrialized countries throughout the world.

How do I develop cardiovascular-respiratory fitness?

The best activities for improving the function of the CVR system are those that are continuous, rhythmical and aerobic in nature and can be sustained for over 20 minutes or more. Walking and jogging are the easiest exercises with which to begin. Bicycling, swimming and other continuous exertions also can provide an adequate stimulus for developing CVR fitness. Three variables affect attaining CVR fitness: intensity, duration and frequency.

How hard should I exercise?

Intensity refers to how stressful an exercise is to the CVR system. Most individuals want to know how fast to walk, jog, swim or exercise for the body to get stronger and improve its health. Exercise physiologists have determined how fast the heart should beat while exercising in order to produce a training effect. A person's heart rate is normally proportional to the amount of stress placed upon the body.

Ways of exercising to elevate the heart beat to a desirable threshold intensity include walking briskly, jogging, swimming, cycling or playing a vigorous game such as tennis or racquetball. To determine the desired intensity or rate of your heart beat, record your pulse beat immediately after exercising for four or five minutes. If your heart rate is below the desired rate, then speed up your method of exercise. You may need to walk or jog a little faster to cause your heart rate to rise with increased intensity until it reaches a steady state (a condition in which the CVR system can supply enough oxygen to the muscles so that they can create enough energy to do the exercise work). If your heart rate is higher than the threshold intensity, you may want to slow down your exercise pace. Slowing down is unnecessary if you desire to increase your CVR fitness to a higher degree. The higher the intensity, the greater the increase in CVR endurance.

The best place on the body to record the pulse rate is at the radial artery of the wrist just below the thumb. To determine the number of heart beats per minute, apply pressure with the fingers on the wrist, count the number of beats in 15 seconds, and multiply by four.

How long should I exercise?

The duration of an exercise also is very important in improving the cardiovascular functions in the body. The duration of an exercise should be proportionate to your present level of cardiovascular fitness. If you are highly fit, you should exercise longer. This longer duration will increase cardiovascular fitness to your optimum level. Conversely, if your fitness is low, you should exercise for a shorter time or until you are able to increase your time slowly and progressively. As you get stronger, you can safely increase your duration without unduly stressing the cardiovascular system. Depending on your present fitness level, try to exercise continuously for 20 to 40 minutes.

How often should I exercise?

Determining the necessary frequency of exercise also is important. The key to safe exercising is to develop consistency. Make an effort to exercise at least three times a week, preferably four to five times. Find a specific time of day for exercising and stick with it. Guard this precious time from any outside interference.

Here are some benefits of regular exercise:

1. Increased general feeling of health and well-being
2. Higher fatigue levels and greater physical work capacity
3. Decreases body fat and increases lean body weight
4. Increases basal metabolic rate
5. Decreases stress levels by reducing neuromuscular tension
6. Delayed aging process
7. Stimulation of mental activity
8. Better digestion and bowel movement.
9. Reduces heart disease risk factors
10. Improves quality of sleep
11. Prevention of lower back pain
12. Improved functioning of internal organs

How do I get started?

If you are younger than 35 years and in good health, it is not necessary to see a physician before beginning an exercise program. If you are over 35 and have been inactive for many years, consider seeing a physician first. Existing health problems that indicate a possible need for medical clearance are heart disease, high blood pressure, shortness of breath after mild exertion, arthritis and musculoskeletal disorders. Although vigorous exercise does involve minimal health risks for those in good health, far greater risks accumulate with long-term inactivity and obesity.

How can I develop muscular strength and endurance?

An exercise program should include not only cardiovascular-respiratory training but also muscular-strength and endurance training as well. One of the most important health benefits from muscular training is the rehabilitation of postural defects. As we get older, our posture deviates from its natural alignment. In many instances, shoulders slump and rotate forward, and stomach muscles weaken, causing the abdomen to protrude outward. Sometimes the pelvis rotates forward, causing severe lower back pain. Also, the muscles in the hips, legs and feet weaken, causing the skeletal structure to fall from its natural position, which places pressure on nerves.

Therefore, many people suffer needlessly from postural deviations that can be prevented through proper muscular exercises. Most postural deviations are caused by weak muscles that are unable to support the skeleton system properly. On the other hand, some postural deviations are caused by stronger muscles overpulling weaker muscles. For example, the muscles on the right side of the body may be stronger than those on the left. This can cause the spine to be pulled to the right side, causing the shifting vertebrae to pinch the spinal nerves. This condition, called scoliosis, can lead to paralysis.

Weight training has proven effective not only for correcting postural deviations but also for rehabilitating injuries, increasing athletic performance and bringing about desirable changes in body appearance. Weight training is not to be confused with weight lifting, which is a competitive sport testing the amount of weight an individual is able to lift. Weight training is not concerned with competition, but with development of muscle strength, endurance, power and speed of movement.

All of the over 600 muscles that make up the muscular system need some degree of strength reinforcements. Without continuous strengthening, these major muscles will degenerate or waste away (atrophy). An active lifestyle will change with loss of strength. Many people, especially senior adults, have had to alter their lifestyle significantly because they were unable to engage in the required vigorous physical activity necessary.

To strengthen any muscle, an overload must be placed on it. That is, the muscle must be put through more physical exertion than ever before, or it will weaken. Since everyday activity does not require such an overload, regular muscle stimulation for body strength and endurance must be provided. Weight training is an effective means of developing muscle strength and muscular endurance.

A distinction between muscle strength and muscle endurance is in order. Muscle strength is concerned with the ability of a muscle group to exert one maximal force against a resistance. Muscular endurance, on the other hand, is the ability of the same muscle group to make repeated contractions against a defined resistance or to sustain a defined muscular contraction. Most physical activity in our lifestyles calls for muscular endurance instead of muscular strength. Therefore, most individuals should perform muscular endurance exercises. Also, developing muscular balance in all our muscles through endurance training is safer and easier than through muscular strength training.

The amount of strength gain that you can expect from training depends partly on the level of strength that you possessed at the beginning of the training program. If you have no previous experience in strength development, then you can anticipate rather large increases. Those with a high level of strength at the beginning can expect small increases. Normally, strength gains in the beginner can be seen after three or four weeks of training three times a week. Strength gains beyond this point eventually will level off with relatively smaller increases.

The amount of strength desired varies greatly from one person to another. Most women begin a weight program to lose weight and firm their bodies; they are not interested in a strength program. Most men want to develop strength along with a good body contour. Whatever reasons motivate you, begin a program that will develop all the major muscles at all the major points.

Are there guidelines for beginning an exercise program?

- Warm up before exercising. Before beginning any CVR training program, subject your total body to a proper warm-up. Do stretching exercises for arms, legs and back. Walk or jog very slowly at the start of the exercise bout. The time required for warm-up varies with each individual. Sweat indicates that the core temperature has increased and more intense conditioning can be done. Keep in mind that cold weather requires longer warm-up times.

- Cool down after exercising. Cooling down after completion of the main workout is as important to the body as the warm-up. Always reduce your exercise pace very slowly, never abruptly. Do not stop instantly or sit down after you finish vigorous exercise or the blood will pool in your legs and you can faint from lack of blood to the brain.
- Exercise within your tolerance. Do not push yourself to the extent of becoming overly tired. This not only is dangerous to your health but also it defeats the purpose of exercise. Many training injuries occur because of overtraining.
- Progress slowly. In exercise, hurrying just does not work; it merely invites trouble. Take your time in your development of fitness. Gradually work up to your exercise goals.
- Get adequate rest. Rest and relaxation are important restoration mechanisms to your body. During sleep, your body should have sufficient time to recover from the previous day's exercise stress. If you awaken tired or lethargic and your nutrition is adequate, then it is likely that your sleep is inadequate.
- Exercise regularly. Consistency and regularity are necessary for strengthening the CVR system. Spasmodic exercise can be dangerous. Your exercise benefits cannot be stored; you need to add benefits daily.
- Wear proper shoes. A faulty pair of exercise shoes can erase your good intentions to exercise as well as cause foot, leg or hip injuries. Good shoes can eliminate many of the hazards associated with walking or jogging, such as blisters and stress to the feet, legs and hips. Canvas tennis shoes are not good for walking and jogging because they usually give poor foot support to the ligaments and bones.
- Dress appropriately in cold conditions. Most people overdress when they exercise in cold temperatures. Usually, one or two layers of light clothing, a knit cap covering the head and ears, and knit gloves are sufficient. In very cold weather, a ski mask can work to protect the face and warm the air as it goes into the lungs.

- Establish realistic goals based on a formal health, medical and fitness assessment.
- Monitor yourself daily and record results in a logbook.
- Include significant others for reinforcement.
- Have fun!

How fast should I walk?

Talk with someone while you walk. This is a good indicator of the correct intensity of training. If you can't carry on a conversation using short sentences, then you may be walking too fast for your present fitness level. On the other hand, if you are not even slightly winded while talking and walking, then you should increase your pace.

I'm 75 years old. Is it too late to get any benefits from an exercise program?

No! Make sure that you have clearance from a medical professional, but it is not too late. Many positive benefits have resulted from exercise programs for older people. Larry Lewis, who was 105 when he died, claimed to hold the world's record for the 100-yard dash for men over 100. He ran the dash in 17.6 seconds. What will you be able to do when you are 100?

I have arthritis. Should I exercise?

Most physicians recommend some type of slow, smooth and continuous movement as a form of exercise to help stop the progression of arthritis. Most arthritis sufferers have good days and bad days. Start your movement exercises on a good day and keep at it. You may try walking, swimming or stationary cycling.

Can I prevent a heart attack if I improve my cardiovascular fitness?

One of the highest risk factors that contributes to heart disease is inactivity. Inactive people have a greater incidence of heart disease than active people. Cardiovascular fitness cannot promise you immunity from heart disease, but it decreases your chances of incurring an attack.

Research has shown that cardiovascular fitness decreases the severity of an attack, which will increase your chance of survival if you do have an attack.

I have varicose veins. Should I exercise?

Your physician can determine the seriousness of this situation and advise you about exercise. Exercise improves circulation to the legs and can relieve the pressure in the veins. You could swim or cycle as a mode of exercise instead of walking or jogging.

What suggestions can you give me on how to stick with a program?

- Begin your workouts at approximately the same time every day and try not to allow any outside influence to interfere with this time.
- Record your progress on a chart. It is fun to watch yourself progress.
- Set a goal for yourself. Great satisfaction comes from reaching a goal.
- You might want to exercise in a variety of locations. Vary your route if you walk or jog.
- Do not overexercise. This can cause soreness or uncomfortable pain that may cause you to terminate your exercise program.
- Remember that exercise should be enjoyable. Approach each session with a positive attitude. Be thankful that you are able to exercise God's temple.

Note

1. Some of the material in this chapter is adapted from Richard B. Couey, "Studies in Health and Human Services," *Nutrition for God's Temple*, vol. 22 (Lewiston, NY: The Edwin Mellen Press, 1993). Used by permission.

LINDA HAHN

Caledonia, Minnesota

I hated my body. I described myself as too short and too fat. I desperately wanted to lose weight, but I didn't know how. I needed help, but I didn't know where to find it.

One day, a friend and I were commiserating over our excess weight. She told me that she had a book that I should read, *Choosing to Change*. I read the book and a couple of days later told her, "I have to do this."

In *Choosing to Change*, Carole Lewis lays out the First Place plan. Through this plan I came to understand that God loved me the way I was—though I didn't love myself! I was out of control with my eating habits, my laziness and my complaints about my weight. As I chose to change, I found God's will for my life. He wanted me to be happy, and He gave me all the tools to do it. He picked me up when I fell; He never left my side.

The physical changes were obvious. I lost weight, my heart rate improved, and my blood pressure went down. My knees no longer hurt when I climbed the stairs. My state of mind also changed. I looked at myself in a new way. I actually did something that I thought would be impossible for me to do. Now I know that I can accomplish anything with God's help! I am more confident now. I am out and about, not hiding behind a tree anymore. I feel good about myself, like a person worthy of God's love. I begin each day with God and end it with Him. At times, I'm still weak, but I constantly turn to Him for encouragement.

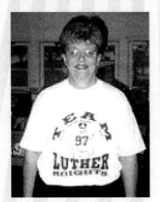

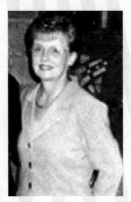

Before First Place

Today

Part V

THE BALANCE

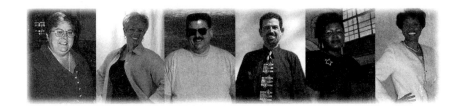

Chapter 17

THE EMOTIONAL CONNECTION

If you feel stuck, bring your whole self to Christ, not just the problem,
but you. Ask God to change your heart. Commit yourself to pray to that end.
It's God's heart to give good gifts to His children.

SHEILA WALSH

Jessica was 24 years old and had been overweight her entire life. As a child, she survived mostly on a diet of fast food and she snacked on junk food. She was never taught about healthy eating nor how to count calories. As an adult, her eating habits did not change. In fact, if anything, they got worse. She often became depressed when confronted by difficult situations in her life. As a way to cope, she would overeat.

At 278 pounds, Jessica realized she was overweight and finally reached a point of desperation. "God has really put it on my heart and mind that I need to lose weight for my health and well-being," she admitted. "I don't know what to do [but] I want to lose this weight so I don't put my health in jeopardy any longer."[1]

Jessica is not alone in her struggle. At First Place, many people write to us and tell similar stories. Usually they are crying out for help. Many times I have been speaking somewhere, and after I have given my talk, someone in the audience would express Jessica's same desperation. Men and women across this nation very much want and need to lose weight, but too often their own emotions ensnare and eventually defeat them.

Is there help and hope for those who struggle to find the connection between their emotions, soul, mind and body? Yes, there is! I believe that our help and hope is found in God's Word.

The God of hope fills us with all joy and peace as we trust in Him, so that we may overflow with hope by the power of the Holy Spirit (Rom. 15:13).

Our God not only is the God of hope but He is also the God of peace.

God Himself, the God of peace will sanctify us through and through, so that our whole spirit, soul and body might be kept blameless at the coming of our Lord Jesus Christ. The One who calls us is faithful to do it (1 Thes. 5:23-24).

What can someone such as Jessica do? Jessica took the first important step, which was to recognize her need. As I read her e-mail, I sensed that Jessica lacked hope and peace for the same reasons that all of us fall into this emotional state from time to time.

BALANCING OUR EMOTIONS

Whenever we lack emotional balance, something has gone awry in our belief system, either about God or about ourselves. Depression is often the result and is one of the greatest struggles faced by people who have a lot of weight to lose. Depression comes because we feel hopeless that the changes we desire to make will ever happen. Jessica believed that God wanted her to lose weight and that He had been speaking to her mind and heart about her predicament. The question was, Did she believe that God had the power to help her change from where she was to where she wanted to be?

> We sometimes fear to bring our troubles to God, because they must seem small to Him who sitteth on the circle of the earth. But if they are large enough to vex and endanger our welfare, they are large enough to touch His heart of love. For love does not measure by a merchant's scales, not with a surveyor's chain. It hath a delicacy . . . unknown in any handling of material substance.
>
> —R. A. TORREY

Most of us deal with a faulty belief system. We have trouble believing that God really knows everything about us and, if He does know, that He really cares. The resounding cry of my heart is *Yes, He knows and He cares.* We need to hear these words and we must believe them.

God has repeatedly proved Himself to me. In good times and in bad times, God has confirmed what I believe about Him to be true. Through the big ordeals of Johnny's cancer, Shari's death, our bankruptcy and our house burning, God has displayed His mighty power. Through the smaller worries, such as having four surgeries in three years, having a bulging disc in my neck and facing tough publishing deadlines, I have found God to be the provider and sustainer of all life. He is our help in time of need.

The Bible, His written Word to you and me, is full of truth about God. If we are ever to be balanced emotionally, we must read, study and memorize His Word. Learning to apply the truth of God's Word and having an active prayer life are the only actions that will guarantee lasting change in our emotions.

FEARING FAILURE

Everyone faces fear at one time or another. One of the most common forms of fear is the fear of failure. We worry that we will not be able to complete specific tasks and we worry over the bigger issues in our lives. Trepidation weakens our hearts, robs us of peace of mind and saps our energy. The nightly news is replete with alarm-ringing reports; and we have a natural tendency toward concern over almost anything that we personally cannot control.

Sadly, fear is alive and well in the world of weight loss. People fear will happen if they do not lose the weight that they need to lose, and many people are afraid they will fail again after so many previous attempts.

At least one hundred times the Bible admonishes us to "fear not." God knows us well enough to know that we need constant reminders to live in trust and dependence on Him, rather than live in fear and anxiety. I have found several things to be true for my own life. In my book *First Place*, I list the following four steps to help you overcome your fears:

1. Choose to obey God and leave the consequences of life to Him. Joshua 22:5 says, "But be very careful to . . . love the LORD your God, to walk in all his ways to obey his commands, to hold fast to him and to serve him with all your heart and all your soul."
2. Recognize that God is greater than your circumstances. Romans 8:31 says, "What, then, shall we say in response to this? If God is for us, who can be against us?"
3. Ask God to make you aware of His presence. In Isaiah 41:10, the prophet wrote, "So do not fear, for I am with you. . . . I will strengthen you and help you; I will uphold you with my righteous right hand."
4. Praise God for delivering you from your fears. Psalm 34:1,4 says, "I will extol the LORD at all times; his praise will always be on my lips. I sought the LORD, and he answered me; he delivered me from all my fears."[2]

Take these four steps today. Apply them to your life and hold them in your heart. As you do you will find yourself more able to conquer the obstacle of fear in your life, whether it concerns weight loss or anything else.

FEARING GOD'S PLAN

Even though I am only an armchair psychologist, I believe that most emotional imbalance comes from fear. This is a crippling emotion that can keep us from believing God or trusting Him to help us. When we are afraid, it doesn't matter how much weight we lose or how smart we become. Our fear has power over us to keep us from ever reaching the potential God desires for our lives.

> Some of the synonyms for the word "fear" are "dread," "panic," "apprehension," "misgiving," "worry," "uncertainty," "concern," "anxiety," "uneasiness," "nervousness," "timidity," "hesitation," "cold feet" and "second thoughts."
>
> —THE SYNONYM FINDER

What are you afraid of today? First John 4:18 provides the answer to any fear you or I might ever have.

We need have no fear of someone who loves us perfectly; His perfect love for us eliminates all dread of what He might do to us. If we are afraid, it is for fear of what He might do to us, and shows that we are not fully convinced that He really loves us (*TLB*).

This verse points to our faulty belief system. There was a time when I was afraid that if I gave God permission to control every part of my life, I would have to do simply awful things—things I would hate. I know exactly when and where I developed this fear. As a girl, growing up in church, I heard many missionaries speak of their hard lives serving God in foreign lands. Many times missionaries spoke of how people in the United States have it so easy and have never endured the hardships of those in third-world countries. After hearing such stories, I concluded that if I ever told God that He could do absolutely anything He desired with my life, He would surely send me to one of these difficult countries as a missionary or He would send one of my children overseas. The enemy used this fear against me until I was 42 years old. At that time Johnny and I were destitute financially. God used our financial troubles to get my attention. I had to agree that being sent to a third-world country couldn't be much worse than the situation I was in. Letting go of my fear of the unknown was the best decision I ever made.

God tells us what His ultimate plan for our lives looks like.

> For I know the plans I have for you, declares the Lord. Plans to prosper you and not to harm you, plans to give you a hope and a future (Jer. 29:11).

Hanging on to whatever we fear keeps us in a prison of our own making. What we dread really doesn't matter. Whatever it is, our trepidation keeps us from becoming the men or women God planned for us to become from the day we were conceived in our mother's womb (see Jer. 1:5).

Look fearlessly at what you fear. Once and for all, expectantly lay down every anxiety at the feet of our Lord Jesus and ask Him to turn your life from fearfulness to fearlessness for His glory. The biggest blessing I have received from the trials in my life is that God is turning me into a fearless believer. Going through many trials, big and small, has taught me what it means to be self-controlled and alert.

> Be self controlled and alert. Our enemy the devil prowls around like a roaring lion looking for someone to devour (1 Pet. 5:8).

Of course, there are times when my emotions get out of control. The difference: Now I know where to go for help when trouble strikes or a problem arises. When I turn to God for His strength and wisdom in every situation, I don't stay in pitiful shape for very long. I believe God and trust Him so much that I have no fear of what this world or anyone in it might do to me. I know that God is greater than he who is in this world (see 1 John 4:4).

When you turn to God with your issues, problems and fears, you do not have to reach for the chips or gulp a soda. You discover a sure and lasting answer in Christ, so you have no need for a temporal escape.

Moreover, when your emotions are whole, it enables you to live a balanced life in every way.

You can take the next step right now. Just turn to God and say the prayer below or something like it.

Dear Lord, I need Your help to let go of every fear that holds me captive. I desperately desire to be emotionally whole, and I realize that emotional healing is essential to living a balanced life in Christ. So I give You permission to do whatever is necessary in my mind, heart and emotions to change my faulty belief system about You and Your love for me. I pray that You will point out to me every time fear enters into my emotions and that then You will give me the strength to give the fear to You. In Jesus' name I pray. Amen.

Notes
1. Jessica (last name not given) told her story in an e-mail message sent to the First Place office, n.d.
2. Carole Lewis, *First Place* (Ventura, CA: Regal Books, 2001), p. 45.

JANET KIRKHART

Mt. Orab, Ohio

God has done amazing acts and abundantly blessed my walk with Him. But my story is a little different. My First Place journey could be titled "Perseverance," because this is one fruit of the Spirit that God has taught me. Since I began the program in the fall of 1993, God has radically changed my life in every dimension.

- **Spiritual.** God taught me how to have a daily quiet time with Him early in the mornings. He has drawn me into a personal love relationship with Him that is amazing, and I have come to love His Word.
- **Physical.** God healed my colitis, which was so severe that I had to go on disability from teaching music in a public school. I took four different medications. My doctors told me that once a person has colitis there is really no cure; the person must learn to control it or live with it. Since joining First Place, I have learned to eat properly and to exercise consistently. As I have followed this regimen I have reached the point that I do not have to take any medication, and I have not had an attack of colitis in several years.
- **Emotional.** The Lord has helped me fall in love with my husband again. God has taught me so much about myself and helped me work through a lot of emotional baggage. He brought me through a long season of loss and gave me joy again.
- **Mental.** Even though the circumstances in my life are a challenge and sometimes difficult to understand, the peace of God that surpasses all understanding is so real.

Over a period of three years, I lost seven very dear family members. The season of loss began when my father—my hero and best friend—became ill with Parkinson's disease. My mother was frail and not able to care for him, and I became the caregiver. This meant living with my parents at the farmhouse where I grew up, leaving my friends and church family an hour away. I had been in a First Place group before moving to the farmhouse, but I was unable to stay involved. It was a stressful time and I gained back most of the weight I had lost. Through it all God taught me so much. He has been loving, patient and gentle with me. Praise God!

In September 2002, I got back on track physically. I heard Carole Lewis give what she calls the Triple Dare—a motivational aspect of the program that helps us stay on target. It was as if God planned it just for me. I lost 19.5 pounds and 15 inches during the first Triple Dare. Our First Place group in Loveland, Ohio, began Triple Dare II in February 2003, and I lost another 15.5 pounds and 18 inches. I am now on Triple Dare V. I have lost a total of 43 pounds since Carole's first Triple Dare and a total of 77 pounds since joining First Place. I am down five dress sizes and can again shop in the section of the department store that has regular sizes. (For more information about the Triple Dare, see Carole Lewis, *Back on Track*, Regal Books, 2003.)

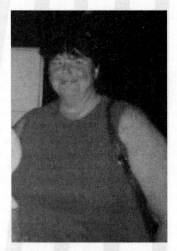

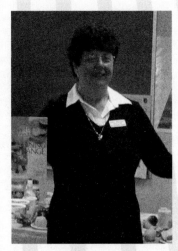

Before First Place   *Today*

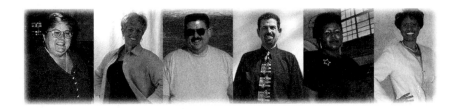

THE SPIRITUAL CONNECTION

You cannot attain and maintain physical condition unless you are morally and mentally conditioned. And it is impossible to be in moral condition unless you are spiritually conditioned.

JOHN WOODEN

Beverly Henson's Journal Entry: September 12, 2000

There are no drive-through breakthroughs. Many times we are in such a hurry to get the victory from God's drive-through window that we miss out on many of the blessings the Lord has for us. We also find that by going through the drive-through, we usually wind up back at square one, because we did not walk through the learning process with the Lord. Guess what, my friends! There is no drive-through window with the Lord. He wants you to come all the way inside with Him and savor every minute of the process it takes to come into the victorious life in Jesus Christ.

Most of us are looking for our own promised land. We hear about going in and possessing the land, but we do not know how to actually do it. How can I take possession of my promised land? Where is my promised land? *we wonder.*

We always associate the Promised Land with Moses and Joshua, but they got there only after the Hebrews were in bondage.

> And the LORD appeared unto Abram and said, Unto thy seed will I give this land: and there builded he an altar unto the LORD, who appeared unto him. And he removed from thence and moved unto a mountain on the east of Bethel, and pitched his tent, having Bethel on the west, and Hai on the east: and there he built an altar unto the LORD (Gen. 12:7-8 [KJV]).

Abram was in the Promised Land. Everywhere Abram moved within the Promised Land he built an altar and called on the name of the Lord. Later, we see that the Hebrew children left the Promised Land and had to return to drive out the inhabitants of the place God had promised to them. My first thought was, What has that got to do with me? I just want to lose some weight.

As I walked into my promised land, the Lord taught me about walking in His promises, building altars and calling on His name. Many of us just set a goal weight and say, "Lord, take me to my promised land." But as we walk into the promised land, the Lord says, "You aren't building enough altars and calling on My name as you go in and possess the land."

I have been on so many diets, and every diet I was ever on had an end. When I lost enough weight, I was done—or so I thought. I know now that this wasn't at all true. In order to permanently lose weight, I needed to change my lifestyle. Before Jesus touched my life and I got the breakthrough I needed, I loved foot-long chili cheese Coney hot dogs. When I would go on a diet, I would tell myself, I can't have one of those right now, but when I lose my weight, I will get one. *I would drive by the place that sold the hot dogs and I could smell greased up onion rings. I would count the days until I could eat some. Sure enough, after I lost my weight, I would get my foot-long chili cheese Coney and a large order of onion rings—and the cycle would begin again.*

Finally, I turned to First Place. That is when I began the walk into my real *promised land with Jesus holding my hand. The day came when I drove past the fast-food joint, inhaled that grease and thought to myself, I don't even want those things any more. I was so excited that I wanted to shout "Hallelujah!" But the Lord said, "Build an altar. You are in the promised land." So in my heart I built an altar and marked that spot in my life. I called on His name and thanked Him for the breakthrough. As my weight came down, I actually began to look for an altar. When the Lord changed my taste buds and I began to eat fruit, I built an altar and called on His name. When I found that I really loved to walk and exercise, I built an altar and called on His name. When I got to my goal weight, I built an altar and called on His name. I build altars and call on His name so often now, and I have successfully been on maintenance for almost two years. I look for those altar moments that the Lord and I can share.*

Beverly Henson
Meridian, Mississippi
Weight Loss: 160 pounds

When Beverly wrote those words in 2000, she never dreamed of the altars she was yet to build to the Lord. You will enjoy reading Bev's updated testimony and pictures at the end of this chapter, but first, a few words about the spiritual aspect of the divine diet.

I have talked with hundreds of men and women who have lost weight. When I ask them, "How much weight have you lost?" every one says something like "Oh, I've lost 80 pounds, but that's not what I got out of First Place. The spiritual change is by far the most important thing that has happened in my life."

Trying to lose weight without bringing our spiritual side into balance is much like being on one end of a seesaw without a partner. God is extremely interested in every facet of our being, but only when we give Him first place in our life can He make the changes that will last. (See, I told you in the preface that dieting God's way was not at all a traditional diet; in fact, it is not even a diet.)

THE FOUR SPIRITUAL LINKS

The First Place program uses four different tools to bring about the spiritual changes needed in our lives. As long as you have some type of accountability, there is no reason why you cannot do these on your own. The four links are Bible reading, Bible study, prayer and Scripture memory. Each of these links has taught me to make the spiritual connection to the balance that I so desperately needed. This balance didn't come instantly but over time, as I practiced each one.

No one link is more important than the others—God has used each one to help me change, and He will do the same for you.

Bible Reading
Read through the Bible every year. The First Place plan is designed so that the reader reads the book of Proverbs each month. Many other yearlong Bible reading plans follow a similar format. Proverbs is a book written by King Solomon, the king who asked God for wisdom. God granted Solomon's wish, and the result is a book filled with God's wisdom for living. (See appendix A for the First Place Scripture reading plan or read from the *One Year Bible*.)

Bible Study
Bible study is imperative if you want to enter your promised land. It only takes a few minutes a day. In fact, the First Place Bible studies are designed so that each one can be completed in 10 to 15 minutes. Learning how to study the Bible has changed my life. Before I came into First Place, I had never consistently studied the Bible. I was taught the Bible by our pastor or by a Sunday School teacher. There is a huge dif-

ference between being taught by another human being and allowing God to teach you through your own study of His Word.

Prayer

Learning to talk to and listen to God has given me the personal relationship that He desires in order for me to live abundantly every day. Balance comes through learning to pray. Sometimes I write in my prayer journal and sometimes I pray aloud during the hour-long drive to my office. Sometimes I pray while sitting on our pier, watching the beauty of God's creation, or while I am cleaning house. The balance comes from actually praying, not just knowing we should pray.

My life is still full of prayerlessness, and usually those times are when I know I need to pray the most. As we pray for our needs and for each other, God hears and answers our prayers. Praying is like my own children coming to me when they were young and lovingly asking for something. As a parent who loved my children, I would do anything in my power to answer their requests, and I still feel that way today. God is our loving parent, and His desire is for His children to come to Him and ask for our needs to be met.

I have learned that if I ask God to give me the strength to eat only healthy foods, He will do it. Praying at the beginning of the day about what I will eat that day is the key to success for me in losing weight. Sometimes it is necessary to pray before each meal to stay strong.

Scripture Memory

If I had to make a choice, I believe that the spiritual connection that has changed my life more than any other is memorizing Bible verses. Several years ago, my assistant, Pat, and I decided that we would really memorize all the First Place Bible verses. In our First Place classes, we say the week's verse when we get on the scale to weigh. Doing this gives us a familiarity with the verse, but only daily practice makes it ours. Pat and I started memorizing the verses in groups of 10. We learned one verse each week and said it as we walked side by side on treadmills at our church. Today, four years later, we have memorized over 100 verses.

Perhaps you have heard it said that Life is hard by the yard, but inch by inch it's a cinch. The same is true when it comes to memorizing Scripture.

I know that God prompted me to drive His Word deep into my mind and heart so that I would have it ready when our daughter Shari died. I am greatly comforted when God brings a verse to my mind in the night or at a time when I start wondering how my family will survive without Shari.

Memorizing Bible verses will also help as we endeavor to lose weight and keep it off forever. Look in appendix C for some First Place memory verses to learn about these four spiritual connections. If you find that you cannot join a First Place group, then at least connect with a friend who may be able to memorize the verses along with you and provide the needed accountability.

I believe that absolutely every circumstance we ever find ourselves in is just a means for God to once again get our attention. God knows that most of us are too earthbound to be much heavenly good. We live in bodies that want their own way. We want to eat everything we desire and then ask God to change the end result. God wants to change our "wanter" so that He can help us obtain a permanent lifestyle change.

The Rest of Beverly Henson's Story: March 2004

In April 1999, I met my goal weight of 150 pounds, and I maintained that weight for five years. Recently, I lost an additional 10 pounds, making a total loss of 160 pounds. The past five years have been an adventure in reconstruction inside and out.

I am single and have never been a good cook, so I lost all of my weight while I was eating out. I learned to make good choices in restaurants, and I even compiled a menu from every eating establishment in my city.

God changed me from one glory to another. I have now become a terrific cook. As I became more adamant about my exercise and keeping my weight under control, I knew I had to be more concerned about hidden fats and calories that are in most restaurant foods. I now own an assortment of cooking utensils and pots and pans—I have even planted an herb garden! I cook to monitor the exact food that goes into my body. I also delight in having people over to eat at my house and serve them my home cooking. Just call me Suzy Homemaker.

Another way that God has changed me from glory to glory is this: When I sat in my recliner all those years, all I thought about was myself. But since I walked through the wilderness of weight loss, God has placed me in the mission field of helping others and giving them the hope that God will do for them what He has done for me. God corrected my "I" sight and gave me 20/20 spiritual vision to help His people walk into their promised land. My focus is no longer on myself, but on the Lord, on what I can do for Him and on what I can do for others.

Not too long ago Carole Lewis saw me jump from the ground onto a picnic table and begin singing at the top of my lungs. She said, "Lord, You have given this girl back her life." I later told her that that wasn't quite right—I never had this quality of life before. The Lord has totally given me a new life. I am a new creation.

As a 52-year-old woman, God has turned me into a very good senior athlete. I have 15 gold medals and 12 silver medals hanging on the wall over my desk. I compete in mountain biking, kayaking, road biking and power walking. In 2002, I was named Female Athlete of the Year for the state of Mississippi. To God be the glory—great things He has done. I always give Him the glory at every race and share what He has done in my life through First Place.

Before I lost my weight, the medical deductions on my income tax each year were sky high. When I was obese, I lived through one medical calamity after another. The year after I lost most of my weight, I had no medical deductions. For two years in a row, my insurance company and the IRS questioned me about my newfound health. At 52 years old, I have successfully made it through menopause with no weight gain. I am a new creature with new health to back up the creation.

I have learned to become a good steward over what the Lord has done in my life. We truly labored together to get to the place where I am today. I am truly fit for Jesus. To God be the glory as I am still changing from glory to glory.

BEV HENSON

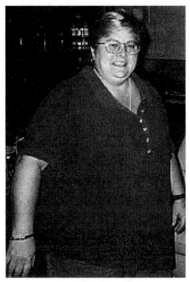

Before First Place

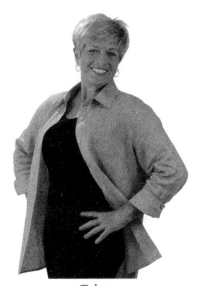

Today

PAULINE W. HINES

New Orleans, Louisiana

I was introduced to the First Place program by a coworker. She asked if I'd be willing to give it a try, and I said, "Why not? I've tried everything else! Why not try Jesus?" And the rest of my story is "His-story"!

I learned through First Place that Jesus Christ is the perfect example of total wellness. His story unfolding in our lives allows Him to be Lord over every area: mental, physical, spiritual and emotional. Giving Him complete control allows Him to give us life, in abundance, before we get to heaven.

The First Place ministry offered me an incredible support system through encouragement, fellowship and an awareness of habitual strongholds in my life—those empty places we so often fill with overeating or undereating. Over time, Jesus Christ filled the empty places in my life. As I put Him first in my life, I found that His righteousness has its rewards. I am now 110 pounds lighter than I was when I started the First Place program. This is wonderful, but the physical baggage I have shed does not compare to my amazing loss of the excess inward baggage I had always carried. God is so good! To Him I give the glory for the life-changing victories I have experienced in First Place.

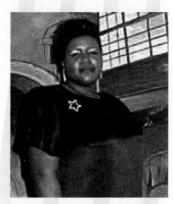

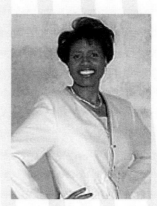

Before First Place   *Today*

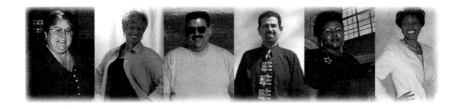

Chapter 19

THE MENTAL CONNECTION

Your thoughts control your attitudes, and your attitudes lead to your actions.

ADRIAN ROGERS

In the illustration in chapter 1, Andrea's battle with the extra quesadilla shows how important our mental balance is when we seek to achieve our weight-loss goals. What can we learn from Andrea's experience? We can see that at the core of the problem that besets so many of us is the fact that the only way we can ever change who we are is by changing the way we think.

Look at what Paul wrote in Romans 12:2:

Do not conform any longer to the pattern of this world, but be transformed by the renewing of your mind. Then you will be able to test and approve what God's will is—his good, pleasing and perfect will.

THE PROCESS OF TEMPTATION

I believe that there are three things that happen every time we are tempted to overeat: *temptation, hesitation* and *participation*.

Temptation

This woman got off work and was hungry. She was fine ordering the steak taco. Temptation came along when Taco Bell fixed too much food and then offered her the bonus quesadilla for free. *Ding, ding, ding. Temptation rings our bell. Our mind starts working out a compromise.* In Andrea's case, she told herself that she could take the quesadilla and feed it to another family member. She didn't really believe this, but this thinking worked to get the extra food into her car.

Hesitation

The real problem in this entire scenario began when the quesadilla appeared on the scene. Those of us who are compulsive overeaters know what the only sane response would have been: "No, thank you. I don't need it. I'll just eat it if I get it into the car with me." Andrea's talking came too late, during the eating of the quesadilla. Hesitation always leads to the next step in compromise.

Participation

All of us have been where this dear woman found herself. We've got the goods (in this case, the greasy quesadilla) and we're going for it! After we eat the last bite, we are at a loss as to how to explain our actions.

The secret to not participating is not to hesitate in the first place.

RETRAINING THE MIND

To bring our mind into balance is difficult, but not impossible. An important truth we need to grab hold of is this: The secret to not participating is to not hesitate in the first place. To not hesitate means that we don't buy Halloween, Christmas, Valentine's or Easter candy when it goes on sale for 75 percent off the retail price after the holiday. To not hesitate means that we do not linger in front of the chips-and-sweets-packed vending machine in the staff room at work. To not hesitate means that we do not go for seconds of anything in the buffet line. Who do we think we are kidding? Temptation is all around us, each and every day.

The time to pray is when the temptation appears, not after we have participated. To attain balanced thinking, we must realize that our minds will continue to think about and want what is not good for us. Retraining our mind requires catching a thought in midair and saying no, before we even have time to hesitate.

> *Retraining our mind requires catching a thought in midair and saying no, before we even have time to hesitate.*

SCRIPTURE MEMORIZATION

Memorizing Scripture is the tool that First Place recommends that we use to retrain our faulty thinking (see appendix C with suggested Bible passages). When we commit God's Word to memory, we replace the lies that we have believed for many years with truth.

I have experienced a miracle in the three years since our daughter, Shari, died. For three years before Shari's death, I had been diligently memorizing all of our First Place memory verses. My assistant, Pat, and I would repeat the verses each morning as we walked side by side on treadmills in the Christian Life Center at our church.

Here is the miracle: Now when I wake up in the night and start thinking about the loss of our precious Shari, God begins to flood my mind with the truths of His Word. Jesus said, "Then you will know the

---

It is not impossible to change ingrown habits if we really want to.

---

truth, and the truth will set you free" (John 8:32).

Real freedom comes when we know the truth and when we live out the truth in our lives. Mental balance will only come when we learn to stop harmful thinking at the point of origination.

FREEDOM FROM WORRY

Another aspect of harmful thinking is worry. Philippians 4:6 says, "Do not be anxious about anything, but in everything, by prayer and petition, with thanksgiving, present your requests to God." If you are a worrier, you know what it is like to be anxious. If we are to be healthy mentally, we must to learn not to worry.

My dear friend Pat was someone who worried—a lot. Pat worried about her kids and she even worried about my kids. She said, "If you don't worry about them, somebody has to do it, so I will." One day, when her son Tim was 14, he was playing football in the gym at school because it was raining outside. The kids weren't wearing pads and Tim got tackled—his neck was broken. When we were in the hospital, I said, "Pat, did you ever think to worry that Tim would break his neck?" She said, "Not once. I never thought to worry about that." Pat said that that question helped God to impress on her heart that worry is useless. I am thrilled to be able to write that Pat does not worry today.

It is not impossible to change ingrown habits if we really want to. If we want to quit worrying, we can quit worrying. Behavioral psychologists tell us that 40 percent of what we worry about will never happen. That is almost half of what we worry about. My mother told me from the time I was a little girl that her mother told her, "The things you worry about never happen." I liked the sound of that, so I just never worried.

> Sow a thought, reap an action. Sow an action, reap a habit. Sow a habit, reap a character. Sow a character, reap a destiny.
>
> —WILLIAM THACKARAY

Forty percent of what we worry about will never happen and 30 percent of what we worry about has already happened, so why worry about that? Twelve percent is needless worry about our health; we worry either about our lack of health or about losing the health we have. Ten percent of our worry is about miscellaneous things that don't amount to anything. Only 8 percent of what we worry about is worth worrying about. And half of that we have no control over. So it's really not worth worrying, is it?

You know, there comes a time when we've got to quit worrying and do something about the 4 percent we do have control over. Our excess weight falls in this 4 percent, but we must quit worrying and begin acting. As we begin eating healthier food and exercising, it is amazing how quick our mental health starts improving along with our physical health.

A GUARDED HEART

Another aspect of mental balance is learning how to guard our heart and our mind. Philippians 4:7 reads, "The peace of God, which transcends all understanding, will guard your hearts and your minds in Christ Jesus." When the apostle Paul spoke these words, he was sitting in a Roman prison. Paul was a pretty famous prisoner, so he must have had lots of guards around him; nonetheless, in effect, he says, "I don't have any guards here. God is guarding my heart and my mind while I'm in this prison."

We need to ask God to guard our heart and our mind. All warfare is played on a battlefield. Where is the battlefield for Christians? It is our mind. This is one primary place that Satan attacks Christians. Jesus said, "My peace I give you" (John 14:27). He said that He would go to the Father but that He would send a Comforter to us (see John 16:5-16). Who is the Comforter? This Comforter is the Holy Spirit.

If you are a believer in the Lord Jesus Christ, you have the Holy Spirit residing in you today. If you don't have peace, then it is because you have not asked for it. God wants each one of us to live a life of peace.

PERFECT PEACE

Our heavenly Father said that He will keep us in perfect peace (see Isa. 26:3). How? We find His peace when our mind stays focused on Him and not on our circumstances. We must get our mind off of our situation and onto God. God is in charge of today, whether we like what is going on or not. He is also in charge of tomorrow. He is in charge of everything that is going to happen to us in the days ahead.

As God guards our heart and mind, we will find that we stop the negative self-talk that is so defeating. If we are ever to experience victory, we must allow God to retrain our mind so that we can not only lose excess weight but also keep it off forever.

As you begin the journey to lose the weight you want and need to lose, it is important that you not worry and that you ask God to guard your heart and your mind. As you begin to think differently, it will be much easier to withstand the temptation to eat unhealthy foods and the temptation to not begin to exercise. Change what you think to change who you are.

PRAYER

Dear Lord, I ask You to take control of my mind and retrain it for Your glory. Remind me when I am being tempted to sabotage myself in any way. If I am tempted to overeat, not exercise or not spend time with You, I ask You to show me at the time of the temptation so that real change can happen. Lord, I want to change the way I think, and only You can accomplish this in my life. In Jesus' name, amen.

KAREN ARNETT

Martinez, Georgia

In 1994, I found myself in the emergency room weighing 416 pounds. Having been overweight since the age of four, I had been on many diets and several times had lost as much as 65 pounds. But I always gained the weight back, plus some. Diets didn't work because I used food to comfort me and to push down any anxiety I felt. I mostly overate because I was bored. God used this medical scare in 1994 to get my attention. Feeling very vulnerable, I found myself listening to a nurse talk about a fat-counting diet. I went home the next day and started counting every gram of fat I ate. Over the next six months, I lost 68 pounds. I still sometimes overate, was not exercising and had many of the bad eating habits I had developed over my lifetime.

In May of 1995, a friend started the First Place program at my church. She encouraged me to come to the orientation to see what the program was about. It was a much stricter plan than what I was on, but I liked the spiritual aspect. I knew that only God could truly help me overcome my bondage to food. With the help and support of people who cared, I was able to commit myself wholeheartedly to God and to follow the First Place program. Over the next two years, I lost 198 more pounds for a weight-loss total of 266 pounds.

First Place helped me see the reasons I was overeating. I found that the television was a big problem. I ate while watching TV and didn't think about how much food I was consuming. When I watched TV, I had a strong urge to eat, so I stopped watching TV—and to this day I rarely watch it. First Place helped me make lifestyle changes that I still keep. Everything I learned in First Place I still do: eat healthily, exercise, put God first and seek His help in every struggle. He is faithful and He calls us to faithfulness. I have learned to trust Him. With His help I have maintained my weight for nine years now, even while working in a bakery!

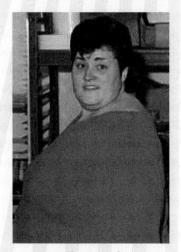

Before First Place

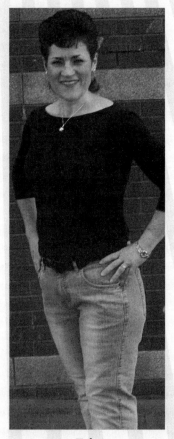

Today

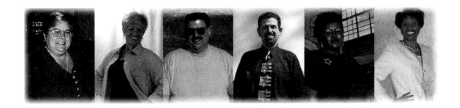

Chapter 20

THE NEXT STEP

*It is for us to pray not for tasks equal to our powers, but for powers equal
to our tasks, to go forward with a great desire forever beating at the door of our
hearts as we travel toward our distant goal.*

HELEN KELLER

I hope that as you begin to read this, the final chapter of *The Divine Diet*,
you are starting to see that there are no magic cures or quick fixes to the
weight-loss dilemma. From time to time, I will receive an e-mail from
someone who has lost 80 pounds or more by following the First Place
program but has regained the weight. They feel hopeless and helpless to
start again.

As I wrote earlier, life is just one series of fresh starts. Success comes
when we learn to begin again before we have gained every pound back.
In First Place, we teach people to give themselves a two- to five-pound
cushion after they reach their lifetime weight goal. The problem comes
when they do not begin losing again until they are all the way back to or
beyond their top weight.

ACCOUNTABILITY

Accountability is the key that keeps the above scenario from happening. Cheri Lasiter, a woman in the First Place group at my church, has lost more than 70 pounds. She stays in our class so that she doesn't start to gain the weight back. Cheri has made some wonderful friends in First Place and she loves coming to class each week.

If being overweight has been a lifelong problem for you, then 13 weeks in a First Place class isn't likely to solve the problem. It may take a long time, but you will be going forward instead of backward. Also, having a friend or two on the journey makes it so much easier.

Personally, I have accountability built into many facets of my own life. I meet a friend for exercise. I weigh in each week and lead a First Place group for additional accountability. During our annual First Place F.O.C.U.S. Weeks at Round Top, Texas, everyone in attendance eats the same meals and meets for exercise and small group times. We weigh in on the first day and on the last day. In 2004, 57 men and women lost a cumulative 221 pounds during our week together. Accountability is the key to our success. We are a team and we all want to do our best for the sake of the team.

The ideal would be for you to join a First Place group. If there is no group in your area, consider starting a class in your home or church. If the above suggestions absolutely won't work for you, then find one or two other people who will form an accountability group with you.

It is entirely possible to lose weight just by eating selections from the 30 days of meals at the back of this book and starting an exercise program, but it is so much easier if you have someone else doing it with you. Your entire family can go on the First Place plan because it is healthy and well balanced in every way.

THE CHALLENGE

God desires balance for our lives in all four areas: spiritual, mental, emotional and physical. This will not happen overnight; it takes time. I began pursuing balance in my life in March of 1981 when I joined First Place. Sure, I slip. Sometimes I fall backward, but one thing is certain: I will never quit.

As you take the First Place challenge, I can assure you that God will meet you right where you are. He may begin working in one of the other areas before the weight loss begins. The one thing I can promise is that if you ask God to begin working, He will.

My weight and yours are no problem for God. His desire is for us to reach our healthy weight so that we can serve Him for many years to come. God wants us to learn to believe that He has good things planned for us and to work with Him to make the needed changes for health and healing in every area.

Truly, the divine diet is one that we can eat from every day for the rest of our lives.

FOOD EXCHANGES
CHOOSING A CALORIE LEVEL

The following tables are designed to help you choose a daily calorie level for healthy weight loss. Choose the recommended calorie level for your age and body weight. (**Note:** See pages 34-35 in the First Place *Member's Guide* for more information on finding your healthy weight.) This calorie level is your starting point for the Live-It food exchange plan.

RECOMMENDED CALORIE RANGES FOR WOMEN					
Age ↓/Weight →	100-119	120-139	140-159	160-179	180+
20-39	1,400	1,400	1,500	1,600	1,600
40-59	1,200	1,400	1,400	1,500	1,500
60+	1,200	1,200	1,400	1,400	1,400

Note: If your goal is to maintain weight, add 300-500 calories to your plan.

RECOMMENDED CALORIE RANGES FOR MEN					
Age ↓/Weight →	140-159	160-179	180-199	200-219	220+
20-39	1,800	1,800	2,000	2,2,00	2,400
40-59	1,600	1,800	1,800	2,000	2,200
60+	1,500	1,600	1,800	1,800	2,000

Note: If your goal is to maintain weight, add 400-600 calories to your plan.

These tables use the best available methods for estimating a calorie level for healthy weight loss; however, your needs may be different. Age, gender, heredity, body size and physical activity influence the number of calories your body needs. It's best to lose weight at a rate of one-half to two pounds each week. Adjust the calorie plan up or down based on how you feel and how well you are meeting your goals. If you are losing more than two pounds a week, change to the next higher calorie level. Also, if you're not losing weight, check your portion sizes—many people don't realize how much they're eating!

CALORIE LEVEL EXCHANGES

This daily exchange plan allows you to personalize your Live-It plan based on your nutritional needs and eating preferences. Choosing the lowest number of exchanges from each food group will give you fewer calories than listed. To stay within your calorie level, don't choose the higher number of exchanges from more than one food group. You can, however, choose the highest number of exchanges for the fruit and vegetable groups.

DAILY EXCHANGE PLANS						
Calorie Levels	Bread/ Starch	Vegetable	Fruit	Meat	Milk	Fat
1,200	5-6	3	2-3	4-5	2-3	3-4
1,400	6-7	3-4	3-4	5-6	2-3	3-4
1,500	7-8	3-4	3-4	5-6	2-3	3-4
1,600	8-9	3-4	3-4	6-7	2-3	3-4
1,800	10-11	3-4	3-4	6-7	2-3	4-5
2,000	11-12	4-5	4-5	6-7	2-3	5-6
2,200	12-13	4-5	4-5	7-8	2-3	6-7
2,400	13-14	4-5	4-5	8-9	2-3	7-8
2,600	14-15	5	5	9-10	2-3	7-8
2,800	15-16	5	5	9-10	2-3	9-10

Note: The food exchanges break down to approximately 50-55% carbohydrate, 15-20% protein and 25-30% fat.

Designing Your Personal Eating Plan

For your personalized eating plan, take the following steps:

- Choose your appropriate daily calorie level from the Choosing a Calorie Level table (p. 223).
- Choose your daily exchange allowance from the Daily Exchange Plans chart on previous page.
- From your daily exchange allowance, record the total exchanges for each food group in the following My Live-It plan chart.
- Distribute your daily exchange al-lowances into the three time periods in your plan.

Here is a sample plan:

MY LIVE-IT PLAN = _1,600_ CALORIES				
	Exchanges			
	Morning	Midday	Evening	Totals
Breads/Starches	2	3	4	9
Vegetables		1	2	3
Fruits	1	1	1	3
Meat	2	2	2	6
Milk	1	½	½	2
Fat	1	1	1	3

MY LIVE-IT PLAN = _____ CALORIES				
	Exchanges			
	Morning	Midday	Evening	Totals
Breads/Starches				
Vegetables				
Fruits				
Meat				
Milk				
Fat				

USING FOOD EXCHANGES

Foods are divided into seven exchange lists: bread/starch, meat, vegetable, fruit, milk, fat and free foods. All the foods within a food list contain approximately the same amount of nutrients and calories per serving, which means that one serving of a food from the bread list may be exchanged (or substituted) for one serving of any other item in the bread list.

The seven exchange lists, or food groups, were developed to aid in menu planning. The individual diet plan prescribed by a physician and/or registered dietitian indicates the number of servings from each food group that should be eaten at each meal and snack. The following chart shows the amount of nutrients and number of calories in one serving from each food group. If you cannot, or choose not to, eat from a particular food group, consult with a physician or nutritionist to ensure proper nutrition.

	Carbo-hydrates (in grams)	Protein (in grams)	Fat (in grams)	Calories
Bread/Starch	15	3	trace	80
Meat				
Lean	–	7	3	55
Medium Fat	–	7	5	75
High Fat	–	7	8	100
Vegetable	5	2	–	25
Fruit	15	–	–	60
Milk				
Fat Free	12	8	trace	90
Very Low Fat	12	8	3	105
Low Fat	12	8	5	120
Whole	12	8	8	150

Bread/Starch Exchanges

Each item on the bread/starch exchange list contains approximately **15 grams of carbohydrates, 3 grams of protein, a trace of fat and 80 calories**. The foods in this versatile list contain similar amounts of nutrients. The bread/starch list encompasses cereals, crackers, dried beans, starchy vegetables, breads and prepared foods.

Meat Exchanges

Each item on the meat exchange list contains approximately **7 grams of protein, some fat and no carbohydrates**. The meat exchange is divided into three groups according to how much fat it contains and **calories per serving will vary** accordingly.

Vegetable Exchanges

Each item on the vegetable exchange list contains **5 grams of carbohydrates and 2 grams of protein, for a total of 25 calories**. The generous use of assorted nutritious vegetables in your diet contributes to sound health and vitality. Enjoy them cooked or raw.

Fruit Exchanges

Each item on the fruit list contains **15 grams of carbohydrates and 60**

calories. Fruits are a wonderful addition to your food plan because of their complex carbohydrates, dietary fiber and other food components linked to good health. They are also readily available, taste great and are quick and easy to prepare.

Milk Exchanges

Each item on the milk exchange list contains **12 grams of carbohydrates, 8 grams of protein and 90 calories. Fat content and calories vary** depending on the product you use. As a general rule, milk exchanges can be divided into four main categories, which are outlined in the food exchanges list.

Fat Exchanges

Each item on the fat exchange list contains **5 grams of fat and 45 calories**. The Live-It plan limits your fat intake to 25 percent of your daily calorie total. One-half of your fat allotment comes from your lean meat choices. The other half is chosen from the fat exchange list.

Free Foods

The items on the free foods exchange list are foods very low in nutritional value and usually low in calories. Limit the total number of calories from this exchange to 50 per day.

30-Day Meal Planner

(Note: There are more than 30 items listed for each meal to allow you to select your favorites.)

Breakfast

McDonald's Egg McMuffin
  ½ small banana
Exchanges: 2 meats, 2 breads, ½ fruits, 1 fat *(Note: This is a high-meat and high-fat breakfast—adjust your menu plan accordingly)*

McDonald's Breakfast Burrito
  1 small apple
  1 small orange juice
Exchanges: 2 meats, 1½ breads, 2 fruits, 1½ fats

Carl's Jr. Breakfast Quesadilla
  1 small peach
Exchanges: 2 meats, 2 breads, 1 fruit, 1 fat

Jack in the Box Breakfast Jack
  ½ banana
Exchanges: 2 meats, 2 breads, 1 fruit, 1 fat

English Muffin Sandwich
  1 English muffin
  1 oz. Canadian bacon, sautéed
  1 slice tomato
Serve with 1 small orange.
Exchanges: 1 meat, 2 breads, 1 fruit

---

1 packet instant Cream of Wheat
1 slice whole-wheat toast
1 tsp. reduced-calorie margarine
1 c. nonfat milk

Exchanges: 2 breads, 1 fruit, 1 milk, ½ fat

---

2 Eggo low-fat waffles
2 tsp. strawberry all-fruit spread
1 c. strawberries, sliced
1 c. skim milk

Exchanges: 2 breads, 1 fruit, 1 milk, ½ fat

¾ c. Rice Chex
½ English muffin
½ tsp. reduced-fat margarine
1 tsp. all-fruit spread
1 c. nonfat milk
1 small banana

Exchanges: 2 breads, 1 fruit, 1 milk, ¼ fat

---

1 c. oatmeal
½ grapefruit
1 c. skim milk

Exchanges: 1½ breads, 1 fruit, 1 milk

---

2 frozen pancakes, heated
1 tbsp. sugar-free syrup
1 tsp. reduced-calorie margarine
2-in. wedge honeydew melon
1 c. nonfat milk

Exchanges: 2 breads, 1 fruit, 1 milk, ½ fat

---

1 slice cinnamon-raisin toast
1 tsp. reduced-calorie margarine (to spread on toast)
½ tsp. granulated sugar and pinch of cinnamon (to sprinkle on toast)

¾ cup nonfat plain vanilla yogurt
¾ cup blueberries (to mix with yogurt)
Exchanges: 2 breads, 1 fruit, 1 milk, ½ fat

---

2 slices lite wheat bread
1 egg cooked with no added fat
1 strip turkey bacon, cooked crisp
Serve with 1 medium apple.
Exchanges: 1 meat, 1 bread, 1 fruit, ½ fat

---

1 small (2 oz.) English muffin
1 tsp. reduced-calorie margarine
½ medium grapefruit
1 cup nonfat milk
Exchanges: 2 breads, 1 fruit, 1 milk, ½ fat

½ c. cooked grits
1 tsp. reduced-calorie margarine
1 slice diet whole-wheat bread, toasted
1 tsp. all-fruit spread
1 small banana
1 c. skim milk
Exchanges: 2 breads, 1 fruit, 1 milk, ½ fat

1½ c. puffed-wheat cereal
1 large tangerine
1 c. nonfat milk
Exchanges: 2 breads, 1 fruit, 1 milk

---

2 slices reduced-calorie wheat bread, toasted
2 tsp. reduced-calorie tub margarine
¾ oz. raisin bran cereal
1 c. strawberries
½ c. nonfat milk
Exchanges: 2 breads, 1 fruit, 1 milk, ½ fat

---

1   medium reduced-fat blueberry muffin
1   medium peach
6   oz. artificially sweetened fruit-flavored nonfat yogurt
Exchanges: 2 breads, 1 fruit, 1 milk, ½ fat

½   large (4 oz.) whole-wheat bagel, toasted
2   tbsp. fat-free cream cheese
1   small orange
1   c. nonfat milk
Exchanges: ½ meat, 2 breads, 1 fruit, 1 milk

---

2   low-fat Eggo frozen waffles
½   c. unsweetened applesauce, mixed with
1   packet Splenda sugar substitute
½   c. raspberries
1   c. nonfat milk
Exchanges: 2 breads, ½ fruit, 1 milk, ½ fat

---

1   graham cracker, 1½ in. square, crumbled
8   oz. nonfat artificially sweetened vanilla yogurt
4   walnut halves, chopped
½   c. strawberries, sliced
3   tbsp. wheat germ or 2 tbsp. bran cereal
Alternate ingredients by layering in a parfait dish.
Exchanges: 2 breads, 1 fruit, 1 milk, 1 fat

---

1   medium cantaloupe or honeydew
1   c. artificially sweetened, nonfat pineapple-flavored yogurt
¼   c. Grape Nuts
Exchanges: 2 breads, 1 fruit, 1 milk

½   c. cooked grits
1   oz. 2% cheddar cheese, shredded
1   slice diet whole-wheat bread
1   tsp. all-fruit spread
½   c. orange juice
Exchanges: 1 meat, 2 breads, 1 fruit, ½ fat

2 slices reduced-calorie sourdough bread, toasted
1 tsp. reduced-calorie margarine
¾ c. blueberries
1 c. nonfat milk

Exchanges: 2 breads, 1 fruit, 1 milk, ½ fat

---

1 small (2 oz.) bagel
1 tsp. strawberry jam
¾ c. artificially sweetened mixed-berry
   nonfat yogurt
¾ c. blackberries

Exchanges: 2 breads, 1 fruit, 1 milk

---

2 slices reduced-calorie whole-wheat bread,
   toasted
1 tbsp. low-fat peanut butter
½ medium grapefruit
1 c. nonfat milk

Exchanges: 1 meat, 1 bread, ½ fruit, 1 fat

---

1 packet Quaker Extra instant oatmeal
1 slice whole-wheat toast
½ medium banana
1 tsp. peanut butter
1 c. nonfat milk

Exchanges: 2 breads, 1 fruit, 1 milk, ½ fat

---

3 4-inch low-fat pancakes
1 tsp. strawberry all-fruit spread
½ c. fresh strawberries, chopped
6 oz. nonfat plain yogurt

Pancake topping: Melt strawberry spread and combine with fresh strawberries and yogurt.

Exchanges: 2 breads, 1 fruit, 1 milk

1 English muffin
1 egg, poached
½ grapefruit
Exchanges: 1 meat, 2 breads, 1 fruit, ½ fat

---

1 small (2 oz.) bagel, toasted
1 tsp. reduced-calorie tub margarine
¾ c. raspberries
1 c. nonfat milk
Exchanges: 2 breads, 1 fruit, 1 milk, ½ fat

---

2 Sister Schubert (or similar) frozen yeast rolls, baked
2 tsp. all-fruit spread
6 oz. artificially sweetened or plain nonfat yogurt
1 small orange
Exchanges: 2 breads, 1 fruit, 1 milk, ½ fat

---

1 slice diet multigrain bread
1 tsp. all-fruit spread
1 c. nonfat plain yogurt topped with
2 tbsp. Grape Nuts
½ c. blueberries
Exchanges: 2 breads, 1 fruit, 1 milk, ½ fat

LUNCHES

McDonald's Hamburger Happy Meal
    Small diet drink
    Green salad with fat-free dressing
Exchanges: 1½ meats, 3 breads, 1 vegetable, 1½ fats

Boston Market Open-Faced Turkey Club Sandwich (No cheese or sauce)
1 c. carrot sticks
2 tbsp. low-fat ranch dressing

1 c. fruit salad
Exchanges: 2 meats, 2 breads, 1 vegetable, 1 fruit, ½ fat

Arby's Chicken Sandwich and Salad
   Light roast chicken deluxe sandwich
   Side garden salad with
2 tbsp. low-fat salad dressing
1 small apple
Exchanges: 2 meats, 2 breads, 2 vegetables, 1 fruit, 1 fat

Taco Bell Light Chicken Burrito
   Serve with 1 cup gazpacho soup and a small apple.
Exchanges: 2 meats, 3 breads, 1 vegetable, 1 fruit

Long John Silver's
   Flavor-baked fish sandwich (no sauce)
   Side green beans
   Side salad topped with
2 tbsp. low-fat dressing
1 small orange, apple, peach or other fruit
Exchanges: 2 meats, 2 breads, 2 vegetables, 1 fruit, 1 fat

Burger King Kid's Meal
1 small hamburger (without mayonnaise)
1 small French fries
1 small diet soda
   Serve with 1 small apple.
Exchanges: 1½ meats, 2½ breads, 1 fruit, 2 fats

Pizza Hut
2 medium slices Thin 'n' Crispy Veggie Lovers Pizza
   (ask for extra vegetables)

1 side salad (vegetables only), topped with
2 tbsp. fat-free dressing
Exchanges: 2 meats, 3 breads, 1 vegetable, 1 fat

Arby's Turkey Deluxe Sandwich
  Green salad with fat-free dressing
  Serve with ¼ cup canned peach slices, packed in own juice.
Exchanges: 2½ meats, 2 breads, 1 vegetable, 1 fruit, ½ fat

Captain D's or Long John Silver's Baked Fish Dinner
  ½ c. rice
  ½ c. steamed or grilled vegetables
  2 hush puppies or 1 small (1 oz.) breadstick
Exchanges: 3 meats, 2 breads, 1 vegetable, 1 fat

Subway Cold Cut Combo
  6-inch sandwich loaded with veggies (no mayonnaise or cheese)
  Serve with 1 cup mixed berries and substitute 1 bag baked potato
chips for ½ of sandwich bread, if desired.
Exchanges: 2 meats, 2½ breads, 1 vegetable, 1 fruit

Arby's Junior Roast Beef Sandwich
  Dark green salad with veggies
  1 tbsp. reduced-fat dressing
  Serve with 1 small apple.
Exchanges: 2 meats, 2 breads, 1 vegetable, 1 fruit, 1 fat

Chick-fil-A Grilled Chicken Sandwich
  Side of carrot and raisin salad
  Serve with 15 red grapes.
Exchanges: 3 meats, 2 breads, 1 vegetable, 1 fruit, 1 fat

Chinese Take-Out

- 1 serving egg-drop soup
- 1 vegetable spring roll with
- 2 tsp. sweet and sour sauce
- ¾ c. steamed rice
- 1 medium peach

Exchanges: 1 meat, 2 breads, ½ vegetable, 1 fruit, 1 fat

McDonald's Chef's Salad

- 1 pkg. Croutons
- 1 pkg. low-fat dressing
- 1 small low-fat frozen yogurt cup
- 1 c. carrot sticks
- 1 small pear or apple

Exchanges: 2 meats, 2 breads, 2 vegetables, 1 fruit, 1 fat

Subway Club Sandwich

- 1 6-inch sandwich made with no added fat or cheese but lots of veggies
- 1 c. carrot sticks
- 2 tbsp. lite ranch dressing
- 15 red grapes

Exchanges: 2 meats, 3 breads, 1 vegetable, 1 fruit, 1 fat

Lo Mein Take-Out

- 2 c. Chinese beef or chicken lo mein
- ½ c. steamed vegetables
- 1 c. cubed pineapple

Exchanges: 2 meats, 2 breads, 2 vegetables, 1 fruit, 1 fat

Twice-Baked Potato

- 1 6-oz. cooked Idaho potato
- ½ c. frozen broccoli florets
- ¼ c. shredded reduced-fat cheddar cheese

3 slices veggie Canadian bacon, chopped
1 tsp. reduced-fat sour cream
1 tsp. reduced-fat butter
Salt and pepper to taste
½ c. salsa

Cut potato in half lengthwise; remove and set pulp aside in small bowl. Combine broccoli, cheese, crumbled bacon, sour cream and butter; mix well to blend. Refill potato skins with pulp mixture and top with salsa. Heat more if needed. Serves 1.

Serve with 1 medium pear.

Exchanges: 2 meats, 2 breads, 1 vegetable, 1 fruit, 1 fat

Chicken Salad Sandwich

2 oz. cooked skinless, boneless chicken breast, chopped
¼ c. celery, chopped
2 tsp. reduced-calorie mayonnaise
Pinch freshly ground black pepper
2 romaine lettuce leaves
2 slices tomato
2 slices reduced-calorie whole-wheat bread

Combine chicken, celery, mayonnaise and black pepper for sandwich filling. Spread on bread slices. Top with tomato and lettuce.

Serve with ½ cup each cucumber slices and carrot sticks, 1 small banana and ½ cup reduced-calorie vanilla pudding (made with nonfat milk).

Exchanges: 2 meats, 1½ breads, 1 vegetable, 1 fruit, ½ milk

Grilled Chicken Salad

In medium bowl, combine 1 cup torn spinach leaves, ½ medium tomato, sliced, ½ medium roasted red bell pepper, sliced, ½ cup mandarin oranges, 2 oz. skinless boneless grilled chicken breast, sliced, 2 tsp. red wine vinegar, 1 tsp. olive oil and freshly ground black pepper, to taste.

Serve with 3 melba toast and ½ cup reduced-calorie chocolate-flavored pudding.

Exchanges: 2 meats, 2 breads, 1 vegetable, 1 fruit, 1 fat

Quick Vegetarian Chili

2	tsp. olive oil	1	28-oz. can diced tomatoes
2	cloves garlic, minced		
1	c. chopped onion	1	16-oz. can tomato sauce
1	12-oz. pkg. prebrowned vegetable protein crumbles	1	tbsp. chili power
		1	tsp. ground cumin
1½	15-oz. cans kidney beans	½	tsp. brown sugar
		4	tsp. reduced-fat sour cream

Add oil to preheated medium saucepan. Sauté garlic and onion over medium-high heat until tender; add protein crumbles, kidney beans, tomatoes, tomato sauce, chili powder, cumin and brown sugar. Bring mixture to a boil; reduce heat and simmer 10 minutes. Serves 4.

Serve each with 1 teaspoon sour cream and 1 small apple.

Exchanges: 2 meats, 2 breads, 2 vegetables, 1 fruit, 1 fat

Tuna Salad Nicoise

In medium bowl, combine 2 cups shredded romaine lettuce leaves, 1 medium tomato, quartered, ½ cup cooked cut green beans, 4 oz. drained canned water-packed tuna, drained; 4 large pitted black olives and 1 tbsp. reduced-fat Italian dressing.

Serve with 2 long breadsticks and 1 banana.

Exchanges: 2 meats, 2 breads, 2 vegetables, 1 fruit, 1 fat

Chicken Noodle Soup

- 1 c. canned chicken noodle soup
- 1 c. broccoli florets with 2 tbsp. fat-free ranch dressing
- 1 slice Velveeta light cheese
- 8 low-fat saltines
- 2-inch wedge honeydew melon

Exchanges: 1 meat, 2 breads, 1 vegetable, 1 fruit, 1 fat

Skinless Roast Chicken Breast

   2 oz. boneless, skinless roasted chicken breast
   ⅔ c. wide noodles (cooked with 1 tsp. reduced-calorie margarine)
   1 c. cooked, sliced beets

Serve with Spinach Salad (see following recipe) and ¾ cup plain nonfat yogurt mixed with ½ cup drained canned peach slices (no sugar added).

Spinach Salad

2 c. spinach leaves, torn	1 tbsp. imitation bacon bits
½ c. mushrooms, sliced	1 tbsp. fresh lemon juice
½ c. red onion	

Exchanges: 2 meats, 2 breads, 2 vegetables, 1 fruit, 1 milk, ½ fat

---

Cheese and Veggie Sandwich with Tomato Soup

   1 8-oz. can ready-to-eat tomato soup
   2 slices reduced-calorie whole-wheat bread
   ¼ c. spinach leaves
   ¼ c. roasted red bell pepper strips, drained
   1 oz. slice reduced-fat Swiss cheese
   1 tbsp. reduced-fat Thousand Island dressing
  Serve with 6 saltine crackers, 1 cup broccoli florets and 1 cup aspartame-sweetened raspberry-flavored nonfat yogurt topped with ½ cup raspberries.

Exchanges: 1 meat, 2 breads, 1 vegetable, 1 fruit, 1 milk, ½ fat

---

11-oz. Frozen Dinner Entrée

   1 c. fresh baby carrots
   1 small apple

Exchanges: 2 meats, 2 breads, 1 vegetable, 1 fruit, 1 fat

BBQ Franks and Beans

1 reduced-fat, all-beef frank, diced, mixed with 1 cup baked beans, drained,

and 1 tablespoon prepared BBQ sauce. Microwave for 2-3 minutes.

Serve with 1 cup peeled and sliced cucumber tossed with 1 tablespoon lite Italian dressing and 1 cup cantaloupe cubes.

Exchanges: 2 meats, 2 breads, 1 vegetable, 1 fruit, 1 fat

Sliced-Egg Sandwich

2 slices diet whole-wheat bread	2 tomato slices
1 hard-boiled egg, sliced	2 tsp. low-fat mayonnaise
¼ c. watercress leaves	

Serve with ½ cup each carrot and celery sticks and a 3x2-inch wedge of watermelon.

Exchanges: 1 meat, 1 bread, 1 vegetable, 1 fruit, 1 fat

Chicken Patty Melt

2 slices whole-grain bread, toasted and topped with 1 ounce canned white chicken meat, drained and mixed with 2 teaspoons reduced-fat mayonnaise and 1 ounce shredded part-skim mozzarella cheese. Broil open-faced until bubbly.

Serve with 1 cup celery sticks, 1 tablespoon fat-free ranch dressing and 1 medium apple.

Exchanges: 2 meats, 2 breads, 1 vegetable, 1 fruit, 1 fat

Veggie Pizza

1 6-inch flat pita bread	¼ cup prepared chunky-style Spaghetti sauce
¼ cup carrots, shredded	
¼ cup broccoli florets	8 turkey pepperoni slices
¼ cup tomatoes, diced	1 oz. part-skim mozzarella, shredded

Preheat oven to 450° F. Place the bread on a cookie sheet. Spread the sauce on top of the bread. Layer with remaining ingredients, finishing with the cheese. Bake 8-10 minutes or until cheese is melted and bubbly.

Serve with 1 small orange.

Exchanges: 2 meats, 2 breads, 1½ vegetables, 1 fruit, 1 fat

Veggie Cheese Quesadillas

    Nonstick cooking spray
2   6-inch nonfat flour tortillas
2   oz. reduced-fat Colby
    Jack cheese, grated
1   tbsp. reduced-fat sour cream

½   cup frozen broccoli florets,
    cooked
¼   cup mushrooms, sliced
¼   cup salsa

Coat a nonstick skillet with cooking spray and heat. Put one tortilla in pan and sprinkle with cheese. Place broccoli and mushrooms on top of cheese. Cover with the second tortilla and brown on both sides. Remove from the pan and let sit a minute. Slice and serve with sour cream and salsa.

Serve with 1 cup carrot sticks and ½ cup sliced peaches in own juice.
Exchanges: 2 meats, 2 breads, 2 vegetables, 1 fruit, 1 fat

Grilled Turkey and Cheese Sandwich

1½ oz. slice cooked turkey breast
2   slices whole-wheat diet bread
1   tsp. low-fat mayonnaise

1   tsp. mustard
½   oz. slice Swiss cheese
    Butter-flavored nonstick
    cooking spray

Preheat skillet; coat with cooking spray. Spread mayonnaise and mustard on bread; layer with turkey and cheese. Grill sandwich over medium heat until bread is lightly browned on both sides and cheese is melted, turning occasionally. Combine tomato and cucumber in small bowl; drizzle with dressing prior to serving.

Serve with Cucumber and Tomato Salad drizzled with 1 tablespoon Balsamic Vinaigrette and 1 ounce reduced-fat pretzels.
Exchanges: 2 meats, 2 breads, 1 vegetable, 1 fat

Chicken Fajita

1½ oz. cooked chicken, shredded
¼   c. onion, diced
¼   c. bell pepper, diced
¼   c. salsa

1   tbsp. fat-free sour cream
1   10-in. low-fat flour tortilla
¼   oz. Colby cheese, shredded
    Nonstick cooking spray

In skillet coated with cooking spray, sauté onions and peppers for 1 minute; add chicken and heat thoroughly. In small bowl, combine salsa and sour cream; mix well. Fill tortilla with chicken; top with cheese. Heat in microwave, if desired, and serve with creamy salsa.

Serve with 1 cup canned tropical mixed fruit.

Exchanges: 2 meats, 2 breads, 1½ vegetables, 1 fruit, 1 fat

Stuffed Sweet Potato

1 6-oz. baked sweet potato
2 oz. lean ham, diced
1 tsp. reduced-fat margarine
1 tbsp. raisins
   Dash cinnamon

Serve with 1 cup steamed asparagus spears drizzled with 1 tablespoon Balsamic Vinaigrette.

Exchanges: 2 meats, 2 breads, 2 vegetables, ½ fruit, 1 fat

Lean Cuisine Lasagna with Meat Sauce

Served with 1 3-inch slice toasted French bread and spinach salad:
¼ c. sliced mushrooms
2 tbsp. reduced-fat French dressing
   Toss spinach with mushrooms and dressing.

Exchanges: 2 meats, 2 breads, 1 vegetable, 1 fat

DINNERS

Eating out at Chinese Restaurant

Single serving egg-drop or wonton soup

Appetizer-size beef and broccoli or chicken lettuce wraps (or split-entrée version)

½ c. steamed or brown rice

Approximate Exchanges: 2 to 3 meats, 2 breads, 1 to 2 vegetables, 1 to 2 fats

Eating Out at Italian Restaurant

Small Caesar or house salad with reduced-fat dressing on the side

Split entrée of chicken piccata or chicken marsala

1 c. steamed vegetables

1½ c. pasta with marinara sauce

Approximate Exchanges: 3 to 4 meats, 2 to 3 breads, 2 vegetables, 2 fats

---

Mexican Restaurant Fajitas

½ order chicken or steak fajitas

2 flour tortillas

½ c. refried beans

½ c. salsa

1 tsp. sour cream

Exchanges: 3 to 4 meats, 3 breads, 2 vegetables, 2 fats

Outback Steakhouse Griller

Chicken-and-veggie or shrimp-and-veggie griller meal, with

House side salad and

2 tbsp. low-fat salad dressing

Exchanges: (for chicken) 4 meats, 2 breads, 2 vegetables, 2 fats;
(for shrimp) 2 meats, 2 breads, 2 vegetables, 2 fats

Pizza Hut Supreme Thin Crust Pizza

2 medium slices

Serve with 2 cups tossed salad with 2 tablespoons fat-free dressing and 1 apple.

Exchanges: 3 meats, 3 breads, 2 vegetables, 1 fruit, 2 fats

Taco Bell Chicken Fajita

Green salad with veggies and reduced-fat dressing

Serve with 3 tablespoons salsa, 1 teaspoon reduced-fat sour cream and 1 medium apple.

Exchanges: 2 meats, 3 breads, 1 vegetable, 1 fruit, 2 fats

Seafood Restaurant Dinner

   Broiled or grilled seafood restaurant seafood entrée (lunch-sized portion, sauce on the side)

   ½ c. rice
   ½ c. steamed or grilled vegetables
   2 c. salad
   2 tbsp. low-fat dressing (on the side)

Exchanges: 3 meats, 2 breads, 2 vegetables, 2 fats

10-Ounce Lean Cuisine Cheese Lasagna with
Chicken Scaloppini Entrée

   Serve with 1 cup spinach salad, with sliced tomatoes, sliced mushrooms, 1 teaspoon Bacon Bits and 2 tablespoons reduced-fat French salad dressing, and 4 saltine crackers.

Exchanges: 2½ meats, 2 breads, 2 vegetables, 1 fat

BBQ Steak Kabobs

   1¼ lbs. boneless round- or top-sirloin
        steaks, cut into 2-in. pieces
   2 tbsp. plus 2 tsp. ketchup
   1 tbsp. light molasses
   1 tbsp. plus 1 tsp. Worcestershire sauce
   2 tsp. spicy brown mustard
   2 tsp. grated onion
   4 slices French bread, cut ½ in. thick, toasted and hot
   1 garlic clove, halved

Preheat grill to medium. In large bowl, combine ketchup, molasses, Worcestershire, mustard and onion; season with salt to taste. Add meat; toss to coat well. Thread steak chunks onto long skewers; grill to desired doneness (10 minutes for medium rare) turning occasionally and brushing with sauce. While skewers are cooking, toast French bread. Lightly rub one side of hot toasted bread with cut side of garlic clove. Serves 4.

   Serve each with 1 cup grilled vegetables and 1 cup roasted potatoes.

Exchanges: 3 meats, 2 breads, 2 vegetables, 1 fat

Spaghetti Carbonara

    6 oz. uncooked spaghetti noodles
    1 tsp. vegetable oil
    1 medium onion, chopped
    ⅔ c. reduced-sodium chicken broth
    3 c. sliced mushrooms
    8 oz. lean Canadian bacon, thinly sliced into strips
    1 c. frozen peas
    1 oz. freshly grated Parmesan cheese
    2 tbsp. reduced-fat sour cream
       Freshly ground black pepper
       Additional Parmesan cheese for garnish (optional)
       Nonstick cooking spray

Cook spaghetti noodles according to package directions, omitting salt
and fat; drain. Return to pot; toss with oil to prevent sticking. Set
aside. Coat large, nonstick skillet with cooking spray. Sauté onion over
medium-high heat until tender. Add broth; bring to a boil. Add mushrooms; cook 4 to 5 minutes, stirring frequently. Add bacon strips.
Cook additional 2 to 3 minutes; add peas. When heated through,
remove from heat. Stir in cheese and sour cream. Garnish each serving
with pepper and fresh Parmesan. Serves 4.

    Serve each with 1 cup green salad, 2 tablespoons low-fat dressing
and a 1-ounce slice of toasted French bread.
Exchanges: 2½ meats, 2½ breads, 1 vegetable, 1 fat

Southwestern Snapper

    1½ lbs. snapper fillets, cut into 4 6-oz. portions
    ¼   c. lime juice
    ½   c. egg substitute
    1   c. finely crushed ranch-flavored
        tortilla chips
    1   c. chunky salsa
    ¼   c. chopped fresh cilantro
        Nonstick cooking spray

Preheat oven to 450° F. Rinse fillets with cold water and pat dry with paper towels. Combine lime juice and egg substitute in shallow dish. Place tortilla crumbs in separate dish. Dip each fillet into egg mixture; press into seasoned crumbs to coat. Place on baking sheet coated with cooking spray and sprinkle with any remaining crumbs. Bake 10 to 12 minutes or until fish flakes with fork. Top each fillet with ¼ cup salsa and garnish with cilantro. Serves 4.

Exchanges: 3 meats, 2 breads, 1 vegetable, 1 fat

Pork Chops with Cherry Sauce

- 4   4-oz. boneless, center-cut pork chops, trimmed of fat
- ½   tsp. garlic salt
- ½   tsp. ground pepper
- 1   16-oz. bag frozen dark red pitted cherries, thawed and drained
- ¾   tsp. dried leaf oregano, crushed
- ½   tsp. ground nutmeg
- ½   tsp. balsamic vinegar
- ½   c. red grape juice
  Nonstick cooking spray

Coat a large skillet with nonstick cooking spray. Coat pork chops evenly on both sides with garlic and pepper. Arrange in preheated skillet and brown well on both sides over medium heat. Combine grape juice, vinegar, remaining seasonings and half of cherries in blender. Puree and pour over pork chops in skillet. Sprinkle remaining cherries over top; then reduce heat. Cover and simmer 10 minutes. Serves 4.

Serve each immediately with ⅓ cup cooked brown rice, 6 to 8 steamed asparagus spears and a slice of garlic bread with ½ teaspoon reduced-fat margarine.

Exchanges: 3 meats, 2 breads, 1 vegetable, 1 fruit, ½ fat

Taco Beef and Pasta

- 4   oz. rotini pasta, uncooked
- 1   lb. round tip steak,
- 1   tbsp. olive oil
- 2   c. chunky commercial salsa

about 1-inch thick
1 pkg. taco seasoning mix
1 tbsp. fresh cilantro, chopped
3 garlic cloves, crushed

1 15-oz. can black beans, rinsed
   and drained
½ c. water

Cook pasta according to package directions (omitting fat). Cut steak into ¼-inch-thick strips. Combine beef and seasonings; toss to coat. Heat skillet; then sauté half of steak strips over high heat 1 to 2 minutes, or until no longer pink. Remove from skillet with a slotted spoon; set aside. Sauté remaining half in same manner. Add pasta, salsa, beans and water to pan; cook 4 to 5 minutes over medium heat. Combine with beef in serving bowl and garnish as desired. Serves 4.

Serve each with salad of cucumbers and peppers, tossed with reduced-fat dressing and 1 kiwi.

Exchanges: 3 meats, 2½ breads, 1½ vegetable, 1 fruit, 1 fat

Stouffer's 9⅛-oz. Lean Cuisine Cheese Cannelloni

Prepare as directed. Serves 1.

Serve with 1 slice garlic breadstick and 1 serving *Sautéed Greens*.

Exchanges: 1½ meats, 2½ breads, 2 vegetables, 1 fat

Sautéed Greens

2 tsp. olive oil
1 medium onion, diced
1 large bunch fresh greens (kale, collards, turnips or mustard greens), washed, cleaned and chopped (or 1 lb. frozen, thawed)
¼ c. vegetable broth
1 tbsp. balsamic vinegar

Sauté onion in large skillet over medium heat until tender. Add chopped greens, broth and vinegar; continue to sauté 8 to 10 minutes or until tender. Serves 4.

Exchanges: 1 vegetable

Broccoli "Beef" Stir-Fry

2	soy-protein patties	1	c. condensed tomato soup
2	tsp. vegetable oil, divided	1	tbsp. cider vinegar
2	c. broccoli florets	1	tsp. soy sauce
¼	tsp. ground ginger	1½	c. hot cooked brown rice
1	garlic clove, minced		

Slice soy patties into ½-inch strips. Preheat medium-sized nonstick skillet; then add 1 teaspoon oil and stir-fry soy strips over high heat 1 minute or until browned. Once browned, remove from skillet and set aside. Reduce heat; add remaining oil and stir-fry broccoli florets until tender-crisp. Stir in ginger, garlic, soup, vinegar and soy sauce; heat to boiling. Stir in soy strips; heat through and serve over rice. Serves 2.

Serve each with 1 serving *Collard Greens with Tomatoes*.
Exchanges: 2½ meats, 3 breads, 2 vegetables, 1 fat

Collard Greens with Tomatoes

1	large bunch collard greens, stems and ribs removed
1	tbsp. olive oil
2	garlic cloves, chopped
1	28-oz. can diced tomatoes
1	tsp. salt
1	tsp. oregano
4	oz. reduced-fat cheddar cheese, shredded

Bring large pot of water to rolling boil; add greens and cook 10 minutes or until tender. Drain and roughly chop; set aside. Heat oil in large skillet; add garlic and sauté 1 minute. Add greens, tomatoes, salt and oregano; cook 4 to 5 minutes more. Top with shredded cheese prior to serving. Serves 4.
Exchanges: 1 meat, 1 vegetable, ½ fat

Crock-Pot Chicken Stew

2	c. water	½	c. chopped onion
4	4-oz. boneless, skinless chicken breasts, cut into chunks	⅛	tsp. garlic powder
		1	bay leaf
		½	tsp. crushed dry leaf basil

1 16-oz. can navy beans, drained	¼ tsp. crushed dry leaf oregano
1 16-oz. can low-sodium stewed tomatoes	¼ tsp. paprika
	1 tsp. low-sodium instant chicken or beef boullion
½ c. thinly sliced celery	1½ c. diced carrot

Combine all ingredients in Crock-Pot; cook on low heat 8 to 10 hours. Discard bay leaf before serving. Serves 4.

Serve each with a 2-inch cube of cornbread.

Exchanges: 3 meats, 2 breads, 2 vegetables, 1 fat

10- to 11-Ounce Frozen Dinner Entrée with Meat

Serve with spinach salad with mandarin oranges and reduced-fat sweet and sour dressing, and 1 toasted breadstick spread with 1 teaspoon reduced-fat margarine.

Exchanges: 2 meats, 2 breads, 1 vegetable, ½ fruit, 1 fat

Smoked Turkey Quesadillas

Nonstick cooking spray	6 7-inch low-fat flour tortillas
6 oz. low-fat Monterey Jack cheese, grated	36 green grapes, halved lengthwise
12 oz. 98% fat-free smoked turkey, sliced	Fresh cilantro sprigs, stemmed
	1 tbsp. fresh lime juice
½ tsp. ground cumin	Coarse salt

Place tortillas on work surface. Arrange cheese, turkey, grapes and cilantro over half of each tortilla. Sprinkle with cumin. Fold tortilla over filling.

Preheat oven to 200° F. Heat large, nonstick skillet over medium heat. Coat with vegetable spray. Cook quesadillas, one at a time, until golden brown, about 3 minutes, turning once. Turn again. Brush cooked top with lime juice and sprinkle with coarse salt. Cook until golden brown, about 3 minutes. Keep warm in oven. Repeat with remaining quesadillas. Serves 6.

Serve each with ½ cup chunky salsa mixed with 1 teaspoon reduced-fat sour cream.

Exchanges: 3 meats, 2 breads, 1 vegetable, ½ fruit, 1 fat

Quick Baked Fish

1½ lbs. cod, tilapia, catfish or haddock fillets	1 tsp. Dijon mustard
¼ cup low-fat mayonnaise	2 tsp. dried onion flakes
1 tsp. Old Bay seasoning	1 tsp. white wine Worcestershire sauce
¼ tsp. paprika	½ tsp. lemon pepper
1 tbsp. dried (or 2 tbsp. fresh, chopped) parsley	⅛ tsp. cayenne pepper
	Nonstick cooking spray

Preheat oven to 400° F. Spray a shallow casserole with cooking spray; set aside. Wash fillets with cold water and pat dry with paper towels. Place fish fillets in prepared casserole. In a small bowl, combine remaining ingredients until well mixed. Spread mixture evenly over fillets. Bake, uncovered, for 15 minutes or until fish flakes easily with a fork. Serves 4.

Serve with steamed broccoli and ½ cup cooked brown rice and a breadstick per person.

Exchanges: 3 meats, 2 breads, 1 vegetable, 1 fat

Lite Chicken Enchiladas

1 8-oz. container lite sour cream	1 8 oz. container plain nonfat yogurt
1 10¾-oz. can Healthy Choice cream of chicken soup	1 c. 4 oz. reduced-fat cheddar cheese, shredded
1 4-oz. can green chilies, diced	¼ c. green onions, sliced
12 6-inch low-fat flour tortillas	Nonstick cooking spray
1½ cups cooked chicken, chopped	

Heat oven to 350° F. Spray a 13x9-inch (3-quart) baking dish with cooking spray. In medium bowl, combine sour cream, yogurt, soup and chilies; mix well. Spoon about 3 tablespoons sour-cream mixture down center of each tortilla. Reserve ¼ cup cheddar cheese; sprinkle each tortilla with remaining cheese, chicken and onions. Roll tortillas and place in spray-coated dish, seam side down. Spoon remaining sour-cream mixture over tortillas. Cover with foil and bake for 25 to 30 minutes, or until hot and bubbly. Remove foil; sprinkle with reserved ¼ cup cheese. Return to oven and bake, uncovered, an additional 5 minutes or until cheese is melted. Serves 6.

Serve enchiladas on top of shredded lettuce and chopped tomatoes with ½ cup salsa per person.

Exchanges: 3 meats, 2 breads, 1 vegetable, ½ milk, 1 fat

Hearty Beef Stew

¾ lb. lean boneless top-round steak	¼ tsp. dried leaf thyme
2½ tbsp. all-purpose flour	Vegetable cooking spray
⅛ tsp. salt	¾ c. onion, coarsely chopped
⅛ tsp. black pepper	2 tsp. beef-flavored
¾ lb. new potatoes, quartered	bouillon granules
3 stalks celery, cut diagonally	1 28-oz. can stewed tomatoes
into 1-inch pieces	2 c. water
2 bay leaves	½ tsp. dried sage
2 large carrots, scraped and cut	
diagonally into 1-inch pieces.	

Trim any visible fat from steak and cut steak into 1-inch pieces. Combine flour, salt and pepper; dredge steak in flour mixture and set aside. Coat a sheet pan with cooking spray. Place meat on pan and coat with spray. Place in a 450° F oven and cook until meat is browned all over. In a large saucepan, mix water with remaining ingredients, stirring well. Add meat, bring to a boil, cover and reduce heat. Simmer for 45 minutes, stirring occasionally. If mixture is not thick enough, thicken with a little cornstarch. Remove bay leaves before serving. Serves 4.

Serve with a 2x2-inch square of cornbread or 1 dinner roll and a spinach salad with tomatoes and lite vinaigrette dressing.

Exchanges: 2 meats, 2½ breads, 2 vegetables, 1½ fats

Orange Pork Chops

4 4-oz. boneless pork loin chops	⅓ c. reduced-sugar orange
1 bunch green onions, trimmed	marmalade
2 tbsp. Dijon mustard	1 small can mandarin orange
Vegetable cooking spray	

In a small saucepan mix marmalade and mustard. Stir over medium heat until marmalade is melted. Set aside. Drain oranges and set aside. Place chops on a broiler pan or use outdoor grill. Broil about 4 inches from the heat for about 6 minutes. Turn chops and broil 2 more minutes. Spoon half the glaze over chops. Broil 3 to 4 minutes more or until the chops are no longer pink. Meanwhile slice onions diagonally into 1-inch pieces. Spray a skillet with cooking spray and stir-fry onions 2 minutes until crisp tender. Stir in remaining glaze until heated and add oranges. Serve over chops. Serves 4.

Serve each with ¾ cup potato salad (made with reduced-fat mayonnaise) and 1 cup grilled assorted vegetables.

Exchanges: 3 meats, 2 breads, 1 vegetable, 1 fruit, 1 fat

Baked Chicken Parmesan

4	3-oz. chicken breasts	¼	tsp. granulated garlic
1	c. prepared spaghetti sauce	⅛	tsp. black pepper
2	oz. part skim Mozzarella cheese, grated	2	oz. Parmesan cheese, grated

Preheat oven to 350° F. Place chicken in a 9x9-inch pan coated with nonstick cooking spray. Season with garlic and pepper. Bake for 12 to 15 minutes. Flip breasts, cover with spaghetti sauce and sprinkle with mozzarella cheese. Return to oven and bake an additional 10 minutes or until chicken is done. Top with Parmesan cheese. Serves 4.

Serve each with 1 cup steamed squash with ½ cup cooked shell macaroni topped with marinara sauce.

Exchanges: 3 meats, 2 breads, 1 vegetable, ½ fat

Grilled Halibut Steaks

2	8-oz. halibut steaks	½	tsp. salt
1	tbsp. Worcestershire sauce	¼	tsp. granulated garlic
1	tbsp. lemon juice		Fresh ground black pepper

Combine all ingredients, except for the fish, in a small bowl. Place fish in a dish and pour half of the mixture over fish. Let marinate in refrigerator for one hour. Grill or broil fish to desired doneness. Baste fish with remaining marinade while cooking. Cut steaks in half. Serves 4.

Serve each with 1 cup steamed broccoli, ½ cup brown rice, 1 small dinner roll with 1 teaspoon reduced-fat margarine.
Exchanges: 3 meats, 2 breads, 2 vegetables, ½ fat

Grilled Filet Mignon

3-oz. filet mignon per person, grilled to your liking

Serve each with 6-ounce baked potato with 1 teaspoon margarine, 1 teaspoon salsa, 1 teaspoon reduced-fat sour cream and ½ cup steamed broccoli per serving.
Exchanges: 3 meats, 2 breads, 1 vegetable, 1 fat

Vegetable Lasagna

6	no-bake lasagna noodles	2	eggs, slightly beaten
2	tbsp. canola oil	2	c. ricotta cheese
1	c. onion, chopped	4	tbsp. Parmesan cheese
1½	c. carrots, sliced thin	1	c. mushrooms, sliced
2	tsp. garlic, minced	1	tsp. leaf basil
1	15-oz. jar spaghetti sauce	½	tsp. leaf oregano
1	c. zucchini, quartered and sliced		Nonstick cooking spray
1	c. part-skim mozzarella cheese, shredded	1	10-oz. package frozen chopped spinach, thawed and drained

Heat oil in saucepan. Add onion, carrots and garlic. Sauté for 5-6 minutes or until tender. Add sauce and spices. Bring to a simmer. Blend eggs with ricotta cheese, Parmesan cheese and vegetables. Spread thin layer of sauce in bottom of a 9x13-inch baking pan coated with nonstick cooking spray. Cover with a layer of noodles. Spoon half the cheese-vegetable mixture over noodles. Cover with half of remaining sauce. Repeat. Cover with foil and bake at 350° F for 20 minutes. Remove foil and top with mozzarella cheese. Bake uncovered for 15 minutes. Let sit 10 minutes before slicing. Serves 6.

Serve each slice with a 3-inch slice of French bread with 1 teaspoon margarine, a tossed salad with reduced fat dressing, and a cup of fruit salad.
Exchanges: 3 meats, 2 breads, 2 vegetables, 1 fruit, 1 fat

Old-Fashioned Shrimp Boil

 1½ to 2 lbs. (36 to 40 count) shrimp with shells on, heads off
  2 lemons, quartered
  2 tbsp. liquid crab boil
  2 tbsp. olive oil
  1 bay leaf
  1 large onion, quartered
  2 tbsp. salt
  8 small red potatoes, halved
  4 small (4-in.) ears corn
 4-plus c. water (see directions)
    Ice

Squeeze lemons into large cooking pot. Toss rinds into pan and add liquid crab boil, oil, bay leaf, onion, salt, potatoes and corn. Add enough water to cover mixture; then add 4 more cups water. Bring to boil; continue boiling 5 minutes; add shrimp and continue boiling 2 minutes more. Add enough ice to pot to stop cooking process. Allow to sit 15 minutes; strain and keep warm. Serving size is 9 to 10 shrimp, 4 potato halves and 1 ear corn. Serves 4.

   Serve each with ¼ cup *Cocktail Sauce* and 1 serving *Easy Coleslaw* (see recipes below and on next page).
Exchanges: 3 meats, 2 breads, 1 vegetable, ½ fat

Cocktail Sauce

  ½ c. no-salt-added tomato sauce
  2 tbsp. minced fresh chives
  2 tbsp. ketchup
  2 tbsp. chili sauce
  1 tbsp. fresh lemon juice
  2 tsp. prepared horseradish
  6 drops Tabasco sauce

In small bowl, combine tomato sauce, chives, ketchup, chili sauce, lemon juice, horseradish and Tabasco. Serves 4.
Exchanges: Free

Easy Coleslaw
- 1 16-oz. pkg. shredded cabbage with carrots
- 1 c. nonfat mayonnaise
- ¼ c. apple cider vinegar
- 1 tbsp. honey
- 1 tsp. celery seeds
- ¼ c. raisins

Place cabbage mixture in large bowl; set aside. In small bowl, combine mayonnaise, vinegar and honey; blend well and pour over cabbage. Toss to coat. Add celery seeds and raisins; toss again. Refrigerate until ready to serve. Serves 8.
Exchanges: ½ vegetable, ½ fruit

Steak with Mushroom Sauce
- 2 2-in.-thick beef tenderloin steaks (about 1 lb. total), trimmed of fat
   Salt and pepper to taste
- 1 tsp. olive oil
- 8 oz. mushrooms, sliced (can use baby portobello and/or button)
- ¼ c. beef consommé
- ¼ c. whipping cream
- 2 tsp. Dijon mustard

Season steaks with salt and pepper on both sides; set aside. Preheat oil in large skillet over medium heat; add steaks and cook to desired doneness, turning once (about 10 minutes total for medium-rare and 14 minutes for medium). Transfer steaks to a warm platter. Use same skillet to cook mushrooms 4 minutes over medium heat. Stir in consommé, cream and mustard. Cook and stir over medium heat 2 to 3 minutes or until slightly thickened. Add more seasoning to taste, if desired. Slice each steak into 6 pieces; place 3 pieces on each of 4 plates. Top each with 2 tablespoons mushroom sauce. Serves 4.

Serve each with 1 *Twice-Baked Broccoli Potato* and a 1-ounce dinner roll.
Exchanges: 3 meats, 2 breads, 1½ vegetables, 1½ fats

Twice-Baked Broccoli Potatoes
  2 medium-sized baking potatoes (about ¾ lb.)
  2 c. frozen broccoli florets
  1 tbsp. low-fat sour cream
  1 tbsp. reduced-calorie margarine
     Salt and pepper to taste
  1 tbsp. shredded 2% cheddar cheese

Wash potatoes and prick skin several times with fork. Place in microwave-safe dish and microwave on high 5 minutes; turn potatoes over and cook 4 minutes more. Let sit 2 minutes; slice in half lengthwise. Scoop out pulp (being careful not to tear surrounding skin) into medium bowl. Add broccoli, sour cream, margarine, and salt and pepper to taste. Mix well and refill skins with pulp mixture. Top with cheese and microwave 2 to 3 minutes. Serves 4.
Exchanges: 1 bread, 1 vegetable, ½ fat

Roasted Chicken with Fruit and Pesto
  1 3½ to 4½-lb. deli roasted chicken
     (yields 3½ c. meat)
  1 c. apricot all-fruit spread
  ½ c. dried fruit bits
  ¼ tsp. ground ginger
  ½ c. basil pesto

Preheat oven to 350° F. Remove skin from chicken and discard. Strip meat from bones and place meat in 4-quart baking dish; set aside. In medium bowl, combine fruit spread, fruit bits, ginger and pesto; stir well and pour over chicken. Bake 12 to 15 minutes. Serves 6.

Serve each with 1 serving *Roasted Zucchini*, 1 serving *Fruited Saffron Rice* and 1 wedge *Kickin' Skillet Cornbread* (see recipes on next page).
Exchanges: 3 meats, 2 breads, 1 vegetable, 1 fruit, 1½ fats

Roasted Zucchini
   3   lbs. small zucchini
   2   tsp. olive oil
   ½   tsp. dried leaf oregano
   ½   tsp. salt
   ¼   tsp. coarsely ground black pepper

Preheat oven to 450° F. Slice zucchini in half lengthwise; then quarter each half. Toss zucchini pieces with oil, oregano, salt and pepper in large bowl. Arrange in 4-quart baking dish and bake 20 to 25 minutes or until tender. Serves 6.
Exchanges: 1 vegetable

Fruited Saffron Rice
   1   5-oz. pkg. saffron-flavored yellow rice mix
   ½   c. dried fruit bits

Prepare rice according to package directions, adding fruit bits at the beginning. Serves 6.
Exchanges: 2 breads, ½ fruit

Kickin' Skillet Cornbread
   3   tsp. vegetable oil, divided
   1   c. yellow cornmeal
   ¾   c. all-purpose flour
   1½   tsp. baking powder
   ¼   tsp. baking soda
   ¼   tsp. salt
   ¾   c. low-fat buttermilk
   1   4-oz. can chopped green chilies, undrained
   ¼   c. egg substitute
   ½   c. frozen whole kernel corn, thawed

Preheat oven to 400° F. Coat 8-inch cast-iron skillet with 1 teaspoon oil; place in oven for 10 minutes. Combine cornmeal, flour, baking powder, baking soda and salt in large bowl; mix well and set aside. In small bowl, combine remaining oil, butter-milk, chilies and egg substitute; mix well and add to cornmeal mixture, stirring until dry ingredients are moistened. Stir in corn; mix well. Spoon into pre-heated skillet; bake 45 minutes or until a wooden pick inserted in center comes out clean. Serves 10.

Exchanges: 1 bread, ½ fat

Vegetable Omelet

¼ c. julienne carrots	½ c. fat-free egg substitute
¼ c. julienne zucchini	2 tsp. water
1¼ c. part-skim ricotta cheese	Pinch salt and black pepper
1 tsp. chopped chives	Nonstick cooking spray

Combine carrots and zucchini in microwave-safe bowl; cover and microwave 2 minutes. Add ricotta and chives to vegetables; set aside. Preheat small nonstick skillet; then coat with cooking spray. Combine egg substitute, water, salt and pepper in small bowl; add to heated skil-let. As mixture starts to cook, gently lift edges of omelet with spatula, tilting back and forth until cooked through. Spoon vegetable mixture over half of omelet and fold omelet in half. Serves 1.

Serve with *Sweet Potato Fries*.

Exchanges: 2 meats, 2 breads, 2 vegetables, 1½ fats

Sweet Potato Fries

1 medium sweet potato, peeled and cut into 4x½-inch thick fries	½ tsp. olive oil
	2 tsp. balsamic vinegar
	Salt and pepper to taste

Preheat oven to 375° F. Coat fries with olive oil; place on baking sheet and bake 20 to 25 minutes. Drizzle with vinegar; bake addi-tional 5 to 10 minutes. Sprinkle with salt and pepper. Serves 1.

Exchanges: 2 breads, ½ fat

A p p e n d i x   C

SCRIPTURES TO MEMORIZE

In First Pace, we emphasize Scripture and encourage people to memorize as much as possible. To get you started in memorizing Scripture, here are some verses and the corresponding topics. We use the *New International Version* of the Bible.

Faulty Belief System

Without faith it is impossible to please God, because anyone who comes to Him must believe that he exists and that he rewards those who earnestly seek him (Heb. 11:6).

Therefore, there is now no condemnation for those who are in Christ Jesus (Rom. 8:1).

Fear

For I know the plans I have for you, declares the Lord. Plans to prosper you and not to harm you, plans to give you a hope and a future (Jer. 29:11).

Search me, O God, and know my heart; test me and know my anxious thoughts. See if there is any offensive way in me and lead me in the way everlasting (Ps. 139:23-24).

Seek first his kingdom and his righteousness, and all these things will be given to you as well (Matt. 6:33).

Bible Reading

Man does not live on bread alone, but on every word that comes from the mouth of God (Matt. 4:4).

Bible Study

The weapons we fight with are not the weapons of the world. On the contrary, they have divine power to demolish strongholds (2 Cor. 10:4).

Prayer

Call to me and I will answer and tell you great and unsearchable things you do not know (Jer. 33:3).

Ask and it will be given to you, seek and you will find; knock and the door will be opened to you. For everyone who asks receives; he who seeks finds; and to him who knocks, the door will be opened (Matt. 7:7-8).

Scripture Memory

Do not conform any longer to the pattern of this world, but be transformed by the renewing of your mind. Then you will be able to test and approve what God's will is—his good, pleasing and perfect will (Rom. 12:2).

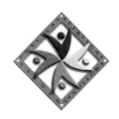

CONTACT INFORMATION

For more information about First Place, please contact:

First Place
7401 Katy Freeway
Houston, TX 77024
Phone: 1-800-72-PLACE (727-5223)
E-mail: info@firstplace.org
Website: www.firstplace.org

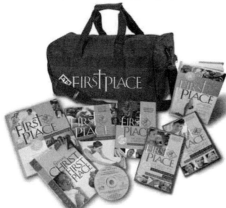
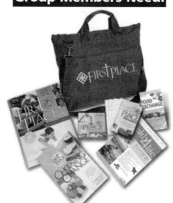

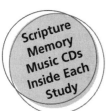
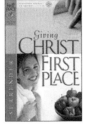
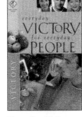
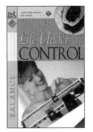
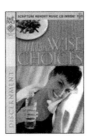
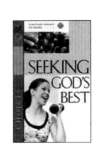
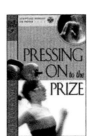
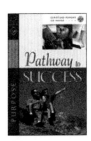

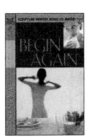
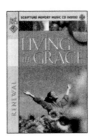
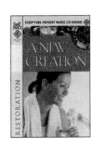